PRAISE FOR

THE RAPIDS

'In search of the cultural identity of "mania" Twyford-Moore takes his readers on a rambling tour of representations in writing, film, and popular culture, and in the media dissection of celebrity public breakdowns. What makes his account so compelling is that Twyford-Moore himself is an "experiencer" and throughout the book we get glimpses of his own life, told with wry humour and honesty.'
Marina Morrow, School of Health Policy and Management, York University

'Sam Twyford-Moore's *The Rapids* is a fascinating exploration of the fragility of the mind, states of mania, and how mental ill-health is treated in art and popular culture ... His insightfulness, intelligence and skill as a writer make *The Rapids* a compelling read. It will particularly appeal to art and culture nerds and anyone interested in learning more about the realities of living with manic depression.'
Meelee Soorkia, *Books+Publishing*

'Sam Twyford-Moore's *The Rapids* is a harrowing and thoughtful exploration of all the crap that makes us human.'
Michael Sala, author of *The Restorer, The Sydney Morning Herald/The Age/Canberra Times* "Reads of the Year" 2018

THE RAPIDS

WAYS OF LOOKING AT MANIA

SAM TWYFORD-MOORE

ÆVO UTP

© Sam Twyford-Moore 2018
Aevo UTP
An imprint of University of Toronto Press
Toronto Buffalo London
utorontopress.com

First published in Australia by NewSouth, an imprint of UNSW Press

ISBN 978-1-4875-0782-4 (cloth)   ISBN 978-1-4875-3703-6 (EPUB)
                                   ISBN 978-1-4875-3702-9 (PDF)

Library and Archives Canada Cataloguing in Publication

Title: The rapids : ways of looking at mania / Sam Twyford-Moore.
Names: Twyford-Moore, Sam, author.
Description: Previously published: Sydney, NSW : NewSouth Publishing, 2018. |
   Includes bibliographical references.
Identifiers: Canadiana (print) 20200254936 | Canadiana (ebook) 20200254995 |
   ISBN 9781487507824 (cloth) | ISBN 9781487537036 (EPUB) |
   ISBN 9781487537029 (PDF)
Subjects: LCSH: Twyford-Moore, Sam—Mental health. | LCSH: Manic-depressive
   illness. | LCSH: Manic-depressive illness in literature. | LCSH: Manic-depressive
   illness in motion pictures. | LCSH: Mental illness in mass media.
Classification: LCC RC516 .T89 2020 | DDC 616.89/5—dc23

We acknowledge the financial support of the Government of Canada, the Canada
Council for the Arts, and the Ontario Arts Council, an agency of the Government of
Ontario, for our publishing activities.

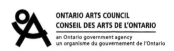

CONTENTS

PREFACE

In 2018, as I was putting the finishing touches on the Australian edition of this book, one of its subjects disrupted the narrative sequence I was completing in my head. Kanye West dropped his anticipated album *Ye* on the first day of winter as I powered through final proof pages. It wasn't the music per se that stopped my workflow. Rather, it was its striking cover – deliberately designed as a talk-piece – that halted my momentum. According to a Tweet from his wife, Kim Kardashian West, Kanye took the photograph of the album's cover – a purple Wyoming mountain-scape at dusk – while in transit to the record's debut at a listening party. The final artwork featured lime green text scrawled across that photo, Kanye broadcasting the showstopper message: 'I hate being Bi-Polar it's awesome.'

Just as its cover perfectly captured the contradictory nature of the condition widely known as bipolarity, the record featured lyrics with direct references to the disorder, including a powerful cut-through statement that he saw the condition as a 'superpower' rather than a disability. My publisher understandably emailed to see if I wanted to update the text of the book to reflect this new perspective from Yeezy, but I was so very late in the edits and so weary from revisiting my own 'superpower/disability' confessions, that I couldn't pull together the energy to do so. How very *un-Kanye* of me, you might say (doubly so, given Kanye's infamous last-minute tinkering with projects and his perfectionism).

This unexpected disruption, however, points to the ever-evolving nature of conversations around mental ill health. An author needs to realize that they can't always keep up and that the static-ness of a finished, bound book can never really capture shifting ground. It can offer instead a record – a marker – of where the conversation about its subject is at the time of its writing. But even that record is never entirely fixed in place. A writer is invited, after all, to talk about a finished work on panels at festivals and in the media, and it seemed to me that it was here, at these appearances, that the real thinking began.

Here was one instance: Sitting on a panel with a writer who had recently been diagnosed with bipolar, who with tears in their eyes, sat looking out at the audience and posed a frank question: 'What becomes of joy? What is elation to you when you have issues with controlling an elevated mood?' I had been experiencing a similar feeling of confusion, though in my case this related to being able to tell the difference between lashing out during a manic episode and standing up for yourself when not in that emotionally unstable state. I had negotiated this complicated field after *The Rapids* was released. The book proved to be something of a lightning rod when published in Australia. One imagines most nonfiction books are ideally just that – conversation starters, provocations, polemics – and that they can act as little hand grenades lobbed from a safe enough distance. They aren't thrown in glee. I didn't know quite what I was in for. Certainly, I did not feel that this was, or is, a particularly provocative book – it definitely wasn't a Kanye-stumping-for-Trump act of contrarianism – and yet, a once close friend emailed me to say I 'did not deserve' – and, more to the point, 'had no right' – to publish the book, making strained claims that I had not done enough work to vet the book with people in close proximity to my manic episodes. The email came out of nowhere and knocked me flat. With its strong language and the fact it hit my inbox the week the book hit the shelves, it only added to my pre-existing pre-release anxiety. I shouldn't have been so surprised, perhaps. People turn. The email had a particular sting to it, however, because it felt like such a keen example of stigma in action. I was hoping to eradicate that kind of response with the internal dialogue within the book, but I had not accounted for people responding without having read it at all.

When I received the contract to write *The Rapids*, I made a conscious decision not to spend more than a year working on the book. I explained to friends at the time that the topic was too heavy to live with for any longer than that. There already feels like there is a radioactive-like half-life to manic episodes – no need to extend them any further by writing for years on the topic, I thought. There are, after all, the ongoing material conditions that you must live in the years after. There are the losses of once close friendships. There are the damages to your reputation. There are the financial implications of past transgressions.

It is, however, possible as you move away in time from your last episode – manic or depressive – to simply forget that the condition resides inside you. Indeed, treatment can provide an incredible sense of stability, but it can also make the illness invisible to oneself. The need to narrativise, or to consider the cultural implications of your diagnosis, can recede too. It has been a pleasure to be invited to write this preface, and remind myself not to become complacent about living with the disorder, as it has refocused me on a central question that has been there all along: what is mania as a cultural identity and what is a psychiatric disability that can disappear from daily life with treatment? If you're not projecting outward, how can you ever be seen?

⁓

In Whit Stillman's masterpiece *The Last Days of Disco,*

Chloë Sevigny's romantic interest Josh talks openly about his experiences with manic depression. In Stillman's typically sharp, purposefully stilted dialogue, Josh observes that he finds a friend's nickname for him – 'loon' – endearing, whereas other terms – 'nutcase' and 'freakazoid' – get to him. Josh likes 'loon' because it's both short for lunatic and the 'lakebird with the eerie call', which might sound twee, but his sensitivity to nomenclature is shared with many diagnosed with this unstable disorder. The same observation about preferences for designated terminology was played more as an outright gag in Tim Robinson's underseen sitcom *Detroiters*. Robinson's father is a mythic ad man of yore in the series and the only other thing we know about him is that he has been institutionalised after having a breakdown in the middle of a business meeting. An old colleague tells Robinson that he knew his father and was actually in the meeting where he 'you know … went nuts'. Robinson stops the colleague and stonily explains that, when it comes to his father, he prefers to use the term 'bonkers'. My wife and I quote that particular phrasing regularly to each other. (Moments of humour are an integral part of ongoing survival.)

These cultural recollections are documented here as a way of saying that the language relating to the disorder is ever changing. When writing this book, I couldn't keep clear in my mind whether to call it a disorder, disease, illness or condition. Perhaps it was all of these and perhaps none. I would type one and then delete the other. I was distressed when my friend, in sending that harsh post-publication email, repeatedly referred to my 'illness'. It was a 'condition', I protested, but then I had referred to it as an 'illness' many times over myself.

This was all unfolding while, in the background, the phrase 'lived experience' was breaking through and with it a significant cultural discussion about prioritising books and essays about subjects from people who have lived through them from a subjective perspective. This was extremely useful in terms of having a way to frame *The Rapids* when talking about it in public. Ultimately, I believe that how a book is framed, is decided by its readers. More than one commented to me that the book was 'quite chatty'. (I can possibly be 'quite chatty' on social media too, and if I ever have another manic episode, I hope someone takes my accounts and passwords away from me, as they amplify the worst of the public expressions of the disorder.) This felt appropriate given a chapter is given over to exploring the effects of compulsive speech in mania. Indeed, the book seemed to take on many of the traits of what it discussed. One of the unintended consequences of the style of broken nonfiction *The Rapids* is written in, for instance, is that some readers with past experiences of dissociative disorders noted having had transference-like experiences from reading the text. This was certainly not my intention (I joked that I had considered asking my publisher to include a warning sticker, 'May induce mild mania' as a way to promote sales).

The intention might have, semi-consciously, been to write a book that read as chaotically and incoherently as the condition itself. But the process proved one thing to me definitively: A book can never be a solemn, final statement on any matter. Who would want to read a book that believes it is that? Rather, here, in front of you, is something restless and often at odds with itself. At a certain point in this book, I question whether memoirs that perform a cultural function should carry with them expiry dates. My thinking has progressed, so let me put it like this: it is my genuine hope that, after reading, your thoughts on the subjects contained within this book are far better than the book itself.

'And I saw that restlessness was neither the problem, nor the solution. Was just the fact. A force. And though eventually it might break me, I would not refuse it.'
Carl Phillips, *On Restlessness*

'Why does madness feel like insight?'
Spalding Gray, *The Journals of Spalding Gray*

WAYS
OF
BEING
SEEN

1

LET US NOW OPEN ON A NAKED MAN ON A STREET CORNER IN SAN DIEGO

There is, waiting for you somewhere on the internet, a 30-second video of a naked man, pacing back and forth on a street corner in San Diego, before it cuts to him clapping his hands together, then bending over to slap the concrete pavement below his bare feet. The sun is slicing through the picture in the way that seemingly only sharp Californian light can. It is the kind of day that invites serious outdoor considerations – get outside, get amongst it! A breeze must certainly be blowing somewhere. Any cooling effects it may bring do not seem to soothe our naked figure, who continues his raging and pacing on foot, muttering something to himself – largely inaudible due to the poor quality of the footage and his own mumbled, muddled voice. He can be heard talking about the Devil. Then he ruminates further before adding, almost as an afterthought, 'Jesus Christ, fuck that shit!'

—

He is manic.

—

Mania – or in its milder form, hypomania – is a state of mood disturbance, typically associated with, and used to diagnose, what was once called manic depression, a completely effective term which has been clinically replaced with Bipolar Affective Disorder. The various editions of the *DSM* – the abbreviation is for the oft-debated, occasionally controversial textbook *Diagnostic and Statistical Manual of Mental Disorders*, which is in its fifth edition as of 2013 – lists the defining symptoms of mania as follows:

1   inflated self-esteem or grandiosity
2   decreased need for sleep (e.g., feels rested after only three hours of sleep)
3   more talkative than usual or pressure to keep talking
4   flight of ideas or subjective experience that thoughts are racing
5   distractibility (i.e., attention too easily drawn to unimportant or irrelevant external stimuli)
6   increase in goal-directed activity (either socially, at work or school, or sexually) or psychomotor agitation
7   excessive involvement in pleasurable activities that have a high potential for painful consequences (e.g. engaging in unrestrained buying sprees, sexual indiscretions, or foolish business investments)

Check off three, or more, of these symptoms and you are experiencing some variation of manic depression in its manic phase. Somewhere on the even milder end of the spectrum is cyclothymia, a chronic mood disorder, whose symptoms are less severe. And it could possibly also point towards schizophrenia or borderline personality disorder. Leave the diagnostic assessments to health professionals, please.

—

The video of the naked man – grainy, shaky and shot on an iPhone or similar – was published by the tabloid website TMZ, a site that spends most of the time in the gutter, fucking with the stars. TMZ reportedly paid around $30000 for the footage because the naked man was Jason Russell. At the time of the video's release, Russell had just spearheaded the *Kony 2012* viral documentary video campaign. Russell's online campaign was aimed at bringing to justice – by the ambitious one-year deadline of 2012 – the Ugandan Lord's Resistance Army (LRA), a long-rumoured cult and guerilla group, and its leader Joseph Kony, who was accused of serious human rights violations.

The documentary – running at thirty minutes, long for a viral video – was developed by Russell's non-profit organisation Invisible Children. The immediate news coverage of *Kony 2012* not only took in the details about Joseph Kony's history in Uganda, but also focused on its creators. The video pointed towards a new form of digital activism.

Within the space of a week, the documentary had gained 100 million views on YouTube, becoming the most successful viral video of all time. Within the space of ten days, Russell was naked on the corner of that San Diego street, acting out of his mind.

—

Jason Russell may, for the rest of his life, feel searing embarrassment about that day in San Diego, but I would hope that he understands why I believe the incident was of such great use, as the most public manic episode recorded. I hope he could live with the fact that this has its own uses in looking at what mania – and, by association, manic depression – means to the culture at large. Too much of this kind of thinking, however, pushes me closer and closer to the first person pronoun. And if it is not obvious yet that this is partly a personal account, let us be clear that this is, in part, a confession, and these are the key elements:

1   I was diagnosed with manic depression as I came into adulthood, following a summer of erratic, ecstatic and out-of-character behaviour, which was preceded by an unforgiving stretch of low mood.
2   So, as a result, I am a manic depressive, and live with that diagnosis and that condition.

When I am talking to other people, there is shame within such small confessions. It doesn't matter whether the person is thinking positively or negatively about this status, I will rake in some minor riches of embarrassment. You can call it 'internalised phobia' of one's own condition. So I can identify with Jason Russell, both sympathise and empathise. But I can't apologise.

—

It is important to note that to speculate on the diagnosis of someone with symptoms pointing towards some form of mental ill health is a transgression. This book is infected with the moral ambiguity of approaching some of its subjects as if they were characters in a fiction, who can be diagnosed, whose traits can be discussed. When I write about Brian Wilson or Kanye West or Delmore Schwartz, it is important not to conflate them with 'Brian Wilson as played by John Cusack and Paul Dano' or Yeezy or Humboldt Von Fleisher, or to even consider them certifiable manic depressives. I do not have the (fallible) medical records on hand.

—

A young woman on a dance floor, who I quickly realised was a former student, wanted to tell me that she too had been diagnosed with manic depression, but over the loud music, it sounded like something of an accusation and that my own confessions, in writing, of suffering the disease had offended her. I walked away from her and left the bar. Later, she found my number and texted, 'I'm sorry if I upset you'. Why did we both confuse each other as being offended and upset?

—

I do not claim to know the mental states of anyone I write about other than myself and, even then, I hardly know what's going on in my mind. I do not speak for others. I barely speak for myself.

—

Jason Russell is such a good example that I almost don't want to go on to talk about anyone else.

—

Joan Didion opens *The White Album* by questioning the appearance of a nude figure, perhaps manic, perhaps threatening suicide. She writes: 'The naked woman on the ledge outside the window on the sixteenth floor is a victim of accidie, or the naked woman is an exhibitionist, and it would be "interesting" to know which.' Jason Russell was 'interesting' to us too. We needed to know which he was: victim of a moral corruption, or just out to be on show. But why not both, why the need for categories in answers?

—

What made Jason Russell inhabit such a definitive public display of mania? The documentary had outperformed Invisible Children's expectations – Russell has stated he was only hoping to get to 500 000 views – and the reaction was initially extremely positive. The video and its makers were, soon enough, marked for severe critical reassessment. Invisible Children's profit motives were called into question and many were concerned about the campaign's evangelical undertones. Russell came under particular fire. The British comedian and screenwriter Charlie Brooker quipped that *Kony 2012* 'looks like a T-Mobile advertisement shot by the Pepsi Max pricks'.

For a film about an alleged cult leader, some suggested it had a cult-like feel of its own. The *Kony 2012* video is hard to watch now – its glossy corporate marketing sheen makes it unpalatable. Ultimately, the product represents an online version of American exceptionalism and an interventionist foreign policy as wielded by tech bros.

The novelist, critic and occasional photographer Teju Cole watched the mess of the campaign unfold and fired off a series of incisive tweets that themselves, ultimately, went viral. Cole used the tweets to damn the campaign as a prime contemporary example of what he called the 'White-Savior Industrial Complex'. In a piece for the *Atlantic*, he went on to explain that 'From [Jeffrey] Sachs to [Nicholas] Kristof to Invisible Children to TED, the fastest growth industry in the US is the White Savior Industrial Complex'. Cole could see it for the moment of rank hypocrisy that it was:

> The white savior supports brutal policies in the
> morning, founds charities in the afternoon, and receives
> awards in the evening. The banality of evil transmutes
> into the banality of sentimentality. The world is
> nothing but a problem to be solved by enthusiasm.

These criticisms were not only pointed at Russell and Invisible Children – Teju Cole also implicated Oprah and other co-sponsors of the video for their support of the campaign – but it was clear that Russell was feeling that the burden was on him and him alone. It would be enough to break anyone.

—

Jason Russell was acutely – overly – aware of what was being said about him during this period. *Kony 2012*, like any viral marketing campaign, relied on real-time opinions for its generative fuelling. It was very much 'all eyes on' – a case measured by metrics. So, Russell himself was watching closely what was being said and answering to it in person on interviews on CNN and other news channels. The relentless optimism of the campaigning was always going to eventually be mirrored back in a negative way. Russell's corporate mindset made him fear failure, but he was also under a level of scrutiny that few have experienced in such a short period of time. That meant he was in a pressure cooker situation that he couldn't quite get out of. He has talked since about a lack of sleep and experiencing racing thoughts.

Russell seems to have been aware of Teju Cole's criticisms and they seem to have weighed heavily on him. In an interview nearly a year after his hospitalisation Russell described the confusion of the positive and negative responses to his campaign, noting that on the one hand he had Bono declaring he deserved an Oscar for the film and Ryan Seacrest wanting to get him to appear on *American Idol*, and on the other hand, 'There were people saying, "These people think they're white saviors trying to save Africa."'

For Russell the competing ideas 'were so polar opposite. So extreme. And in my head, I wanted to reconcile them and I just couldn't.'

F Scott Fitzgerald famously writes in *The Crack Up*, his essay looking critically at his own episodes of mental distress, that the 'test of a first-rate intelligence is the ability to hold two opposed ideas in mind at the same time and still retain the ability to function'. Such a test doesn't apply necessarily to the difficulties of the cognitive dissonance that can arise from a condition such as mania and, besides, Fitzgerald's condescending starting position isn't overly useful, and it is a statement seemingly designed only to be quoted by people who want you to know their first-rate intelligence. Yet the phrase appears in an essay about mental difficulties and related inabilities 'to function', and the ability to operate while dealing with alternate ideas – some self-generated, others not – is a struggle for those with minds in the midst of mania. Teju Cole's tweets go some way to explaining the heat Russell must have been feeling in his head – the symphony of critical voices, competing for attention, the loudest of which must have been his own. Russell's family described it thus: 'It's hard to understand the sudden transition from relative anonymity to worldwide attention – both raves and ridicules, in a matter of days.'

—

One might legitimately question whether Russell's enthusiasm, and his creative drive, came from some wellspring of mania within him. His misguided political actions came from approaching his social justice campaign as if it were a marketing exercise. The heart of the campaign, he said, was an effort to make Kony 'like pop star famous'. This doesn't come from straightforward thinking. The momentum of the campaign left logic behind.

—

The literature of manic depression is made up of a cascade of treatises on its apparent connections with creativity. It is, for me, the least interesting aspect of the condition, but the utter dominance of that focus is hard to ignore. No aesthetic quality is guaranteed because you have known mania. Russell might be a superior example of this discrepancy. He is creative, certainly. He showed a strong interest in film. Russell had shadowed his friend, the director Jon Chu, while Chu worked on the dance film *Step Up 2: The Streets*. Russell and Chu had together sold a screenplay, aptly titled *Moxie*, to Steven Spielberg, which to date remains unproduced. Russell's creative efforts have not always been misguided, but in the case of *Kony 2012*, they have proven aesthetically corrupt.

—

The scandal – both *Kony 2012* and Russell's subsequent break-down – was parodied in an episode of *South Park*, in which one of the show's child-characters, Stan, makes an anti-bullying video, before being warned not to become too egotistical about the project or he might end up 'naked and jacking it in San Diego'. Imagine how you would feel having a singing and dancing cartoon character mocking the lowest point in your life.

—

It was clear there were other stressors for Russell. His organisation experienced an influx in cash through donations, dramatically increasing staff and budget in a short period of time. Indeed, the short film managed to generate $5 million in the space of 48 hours. These concerns would normally rest with the CEO of an organisation, but due to the media attention on their projects, Russell had to front up to CNN and explain how money was being expended. Russell sat next to his CEO, Ben Keesey, in front of a cheap backdrop, answering questions from journalist Don Lemon about the direction of funds within the organisation. Lemon threw to vox pops filmed in Kampala, Uganda, in which one man on the street asks, 'How can they use the situation of war to benefit themselves? To make money out of people's plight?' Both Keesey and Russell struggle with answering the questions. Russell in particular seems frustrated – his gritted-teeth smile seems to say, 'This wasn't how it was supposed to go'. Such footage serves as an archival record of Russell in the days before his breakdown, where the strain of all that talking and explaining clearly shows.

—

Let's talk about talking. The act of talking – and over-talking – feels as though it is both symptom and cause, both trigger and wound. After an interview for a CEO role during a mixed-state episode, I ended up on the floor of my kitchen, unable to move, and unable to stop talking – to myself, by myself – after having spent an hour on the phone in a conference call for the interview. I tripped into the mixed state partly because I had to do so much talking. A mixed state is an extreme cycle of manic depression, in which both mania and depression feature in a rapid, looping succession. A change in this mental weather can take place in a matter of hours. There is a higher prevalence of severe suicide attempts in mixed states – many speculate that the experience of depression mixed with the energy and compulsiveness of mania makes for a lethal combination. Given this severity, the fact that I managed to both apply and interview for a job during this period is remarkable. I am nothing if not 'high-functioning', as they say. Later, after not getting the job, I made recommendations for supporting people for whom accelerated speech and thought are something of a problem when you're asked to call on those skills.

—

There is no mania without its lead-up. It doesn't just occur – it has its causes. His family, at the time, would only describe Russell's episode as a case of 'reactive psychosis'. In interviews since, Russell has made no mention of manic-depression nor bipolarity. According to the *Guardian*, 'His doctors never agreed on a definitive diagnosis but he was sectioned in a psychiatric hospital suffering from what may have been a schizophrenic manic episode brought on by post-traumatic stress.' Russell has said that his 'publicist and the team, they say, "Don't use words like schizophrenic, you'll get labeled for life."' He has not, ultimately, become a poster child for mental illness. I do not judge Jason Russell for not taking up this cause. These were very real things that happened to him.

—

And besides, I am not here to diagnose anyone in a clinical sense – how irresponsible *and* how boring that would be – but there have been some inconsistencies in Russell's telling of his own tale. In the interview with the *Guardian*, he commented: 'I've never been depressed. They thought it might be bipolar but my wife and my mom were like, "That's just not you." I don't get down.' However, later, in a TEDxYouth talk, Russell talked about his high school experience and admitted that 'I was extremely depressed. I went through major identity crisis … and at one point in my junior year I wanted to take my own life. I thought, it's not really worth it.'

—

Uncertainty is certainly the terrain of the diagnosis. It is not an illness with much of a physical grounding, so it occasionally feels detached from reality. It has a heavy bearing on your operations as a human, but there is something light about it when it comes up in discussion or when it is given sustained thought. There are times when mania doesn't feel like illness, when it doesn't feel like disease and when it doesn't feel like disability. In fact, in the experience itself it feels like the exact opposite – it feels like the truest form of health and you feel charged with extra abilities. So, I have, on occasion, questioned my own diagnosis. 'Is this real?' But that is a question that is only for the individual to consider – speculation by anyone else, unless a trained psychiatric professional, is futile. And yet, in mentioning this am I not inviting some sort of open space for speculation from you?

—

In his measured book-length study, first published in 1997, *A Mood Apart: Depression, Mania, and Other Afflictions of the Self*, the psychiatrist Peter C Whybrow strongly asserts that 'mania in its expansion is a public disease'. Earlier in the book, Whybrow states, correctly, that 'mania and melancholic depression are intensely personal illnesses'. The meeting between public disease and personal illness creates the kind of spectacle I describe throughout this book. This meeting takes place on a verge of the human experience. It can be confronting for the outsider looking in, and deeply confusing too. And it is no less confusing for those in the midst of it.

—

What exactly constitutes a public disease? A private disease must be quietly endured on hospital beds and at home, whereas a public disease cannot be suppressed. It often spills onto the streets. There are violent ruptures stemming from imbalances in temperament. In his audacious *The Adventures of Augie March*, Saul Bellow writes, 'Everybody knows there is no fineness or accuracy of suppression; if you hold down one thing you hold down the adjoining.' For the manic depressive, once public, and in crisis, there is no option for self-control. Russell felt out of control and said he was 'like a puppet'.

From that point, someone needed to intervene to stop this riot-of-one.

In an interview on the podcast for a hipster Christian magazine, *Relevant*, Russell spoke about his frustration with being associated with the video of his breakdown and stressed that 'for millions of people that is who I am ... I am that TMZ video'.

—

I am mania.

—

Instead of seeing the second viral video – one that was out of his control, and much more personal – as an opportunity to change tack, and focus on a campaign for more awareness around mental health, Russell and the Invisible Children team attempted to re-prosecute the case against Kony. In the wake of the TMZ video, they released a new documentary called *Move*. It decidedly did not move, going on to reach only around 100 000 views. The new short film addressed Russell's breakdown but didn't delve very deep. Not everyone who has a manic episode needs to become an immediate advocate for better mental health services or greater awareness, of course, but given Russell's previous awareness of what media attention for progressive causes could achieve, it seems strange, and somewhat egotistical, that he didn't see this as a legitimate option – or, indeed, as a redemption narrative ready for the taking.

—

Jason Russell's unfortunate sense of shame is clearly too deep for him to see that course in front of him. Now if you search for Jason Russell on the internet, nine out of the ten top results refer to, or are directly about, his manic episode. This is the way you come to be marked by mania; stained by stigma. But, then, in writing about him here, am I not also continuing to define the man by that single day in San Diego? Or am I doing the opposite: am I reducing the stigma, normalising his behaviour and saying this can happen to anyone but especially someone like me, maybe not you, I mean I don't know you, but maybe you?

—

The media was extremely confused and concerned by Russell's nudity in the aftermath of the event. *Slate* magazine ran an explainer, asking, 'Why do psychotic people strip naked?', which unhelpfully lumped Russell in with Rudy Eugene – the Causeway Cannibal, also known as the Miami Zombie – who had attacked and maimed a homeless man, Ronald Poppo, during a psychotic episode in Florida in 2012. The eighteen-minute encounter was filmed and, inexplicably, uploaded online. Poppo was blinded in the attack, and lost most of his face above his beard. Eugene was shot to death at the scene of the crime, leaving little explanation for the attack. A toxicology report only discovered that there were traces of cannabis in Eugene's system, despite widespread media speculation of his use of bath salts. The extreme violence of Eugene's behaviour suggests he was frenzied rather than manic, but frenzied is just an adjective, not a diagnosable condition. Some behaviours are too extreme to be laid out as concrete medical concepts in our minds.

In late June 2016, a twenty-year-old fashion model, Krit McClean, made his way to Times Square in New York City in the grip of paranoia, fearing that a group of unknown people were out to kill him. Once there, he believed that the billboards surrounding him were sending him subliminal messages. He stripped naked before parading on the top of a booth that sold tickets to Broadway musicals and theatre shows. The episode, as public as it gets, with the high traffic of one of the most populous spots in one of the world's largest cities, ended 'seven days of mania' for McClean. In a reflective recount of the episode written for the tabloid publication *New York Post*, McClean wrote in a clipped, poetic style: '"Express Yourself", read the billboard for Express jeans. I obeyed. I immediately took off my clothes. Being naked, I thought, was the most truthful way of expressing myself. It made me feel safe.'

Is there any truth to be found in nakedness? McClean's body, in the videos and photographs of that day, told a certain truth. His body is extremely lean – his ribs are visibly showing through tight skin, no fat – as dictated by his profession's demand for physical perfection. The work done to keep his body in this condition could be worth considering when looking at his mania. Is the mind neglected when the body comes first? McClean's mind sent him in stranger directions than just removing his clothes. He also made demands to see Donald Trump and cried out 'Yeezy!', the nickname of Kanye West, who within months would be having his own public meltdown.

—

One of the distinct expressions of mania is an increase in sexualised behaviour. Nudity is not necessarily connected to sexual behaviour, nor even sexuality. Certainly, the examples given here defy sexualisation. Russell's and McLean's nakedness stand, almost, in opposition to sexualisation; they are aggressive outward manifestations of fragile states of mind. There were reports, early on, that Russell was masturbating when caught on that San Diego street, but there was no proof of that in the video or resulting reports. But even if he was, would it have been necessarily a sexual act, if one's mind is in such an abnormal state? I am not saying that such a state abolishes personal responsibility, nor diminishes the experience of any victims, but when someone is in the midst of mania where does one draw the line?

—

Increased sex drive is a total nuisance – it creates chaos with your private life and relations to others. It puts you at risk of any number of diseases (safe sex isn't in the forefront of the manic mind, which will take what it can get, any form, any place, any time). It can distort personal sexual preferences too. Men and women become equally attractive, if only sought for personal satisfaction. There are benefits to this increase in goal-directed activity (either socially, at work or school, or sexually), however. The psychomotor agitation runs on and your ego's drive to achieve – to be seen achieving, to impress others – becomes its own strange sexual function. TMI?

—

Do we even need to note how closely nakedness and insanity have been linked since the earliest times? In Luke 8:27: 'As he stepped out on land, a man of the city who had demons met him. For a long time he had worn no clothes, and he did not live in a house but in the tombs.' Poor guy.

—

In a library of medical facts on insanity: 'A striking and characteristic circumstance is the propensity to go quite naked.'

—

Quite naked, indeed. In his seminal *Ways of Seeing*, the late critic and radical humanist John Berger crafts the following observation:

> To be naked is to be oneself. To be nude is to be seen
> naked by others and yet not recognized for oneself.
> A naked body has to be seen as an object in order to
> become a nude. (The sight of it as an object stimulates
> the use of it as an object.) Nakedness reveals itself.
> Nudity is placed on display. To be naked is to be
> without disguise. To be on display is to have the
> surface of one's own skin, the hairs of one's own body,
> turned into a disguise, which, in that situation, can
> never be discarded. The nude is condemned to never
> being naked.

Was Jason Russell naked or nude? One must respectfully diverge with Berger's thinking here, as Russell was both. Russell was seen by others as a nude – unrecognisable to his loved ones and to himself, clearly – but he was also in Berger's sense naked, walking around without disguise. So, it is in this sense that I do not buy Jason Russell's line about not 'being himself'. I do not mean this in a mean-spirited way; I only mean to point out that we all have the capacity to become what he was that day. We can all break. Mania is not, then, exclusive for those with diagnosable psychiatric disorders. It is accessible to the everyday person – you, me, whoever you want to imagine in your mind. The nude can be naked, but, perhaps, only in a state of pure dissociation, when one's nudity or nakedness is not yours to choose, when your unconscious overrides all sense of the societally set standards of dignity.

—

These are attempts then, surely, to make mania bodily, and seen. Nakedness is a relatively harmless attempt at this. For me, any attempt to render the interiority of mania as external, unfortunately, was most commonly expressed in the form of self-harm. Strangely enough, these actions did not leave much in the way of visible marks.

—

The ability to come clean about all this comes as a real privilege. Not everyone feels the same level of safety to take this stand. A friend diagnosed with the same condition admits to being envious of my decision to write so freely and openly on the topic. She says she feels closeted, in comparison, wary of being so public due to possible work-related ramifications. 'It's like being gay in the fifties,' she says. 'It's like being closeted … yet you can also tell when someone else has the condition. You can just tell. You form a kind of secret society like that.'

—

After Russell had spent seventeen days recovering in a psychiatric ward, it was Oprah who finally locked down the exclusive interview with him after his naked meltdown. Russell's fragile reality must have been severely challenged when Oprah herself came to his house to host the interview. Russell sits as neatly as his crisp, light purple shirt and as narrowly as his straitlaced tie. He doesn't take up much room, and looks mildly discomforted despite being in his own house. Later, his wife, Danica, joins him and he relaxes as he holds her hand, comforting her as she gives her side of the story. The overall conversation is, as to be expected of an Oprah interview, mostly earnest. The awkwardly handsome Russell ('the nuts shouldn't be this good looking') tries his best to answer Oprah's gently oppressive line of questioning, and attempts to lay it bare. He performs contrition, but should he? Oprah wants to know the core of the experience, and to transmit its immediate experiences to her audience she goes mining for meaning:

> OPRAH: So what does a breakdown feel like? Because we want to go through the anatomy of a nervous breakdown. Take me through it.

> JASON: A breakdown feels like you're on a special mission … my mouth wouldn't stop talking. I talk a lot as it is, I'm a talker, but this was pressured speech to the point where I would have to go like this [covers mouth with hands].

> OPRAH: Really? To stop yourself?

JASON: I couldn't stop talking.

OPRAH: Were you speeding in your head?

JASON: It was racing. It was just so much. The Twitter feed, the phone calls, the text messages, the meetings. It never stopped. My brain kept going.

OPRAH: So did you go crazy?

JASON: Oh yeah. Oh yeah. It was like a soda can. And you shake it up and it explodes in the air.

OPRAH: How do you end up on the street naked?

JASON: I wish I knew. I really wish I knew. But I want people to know that I take responsibility for that.

Russell takes responsibility for what occurred on the street, but soon enough he offered another reading of the circumstances that led to the events on that clear-skied day:

OPRAH: So when you look at the tape, what do you think?

JASON: When I look at that person, I see someone alone, I see someone who is totally out of control ... I look at that video and think, 'How sad for him.' Your mind is so, so powerful. You know this. It's so strong. And if you feed it with this chaotic noise ... you lose who you are.

'*Him.*' '*Him.*' '*Him.*' There is something within this distancing of the self which disturbs me, and yet one must also recognise that during any dissociative state one really does not recognise oneself. In literature, 'oneself' is not quite the same as 'me' or 'I'. There is a deliberate remove. But it still somehow stinks of PR strategy, and the redemption arc accessible to Russell is made possible by that negation of the self, of the younger version of himself who may have suffered depression, and the acute crisis of his mania.

—

One of the many outward signs of mania can be found within a sufferer's delusions of grandeur – a lack of regulation that trips into megalomania. In my case, it made me email editors and other colleagues telling them that I could do their job much better than they could. In its extreme incarnation it leads to a disfiguring of the self and, in some cases, the assumption of a different identity. The most common case in the West seems to be people believing they are the returned Jesus Christ.

For Russell, however, something really extraordinary was happening to him, and he was, for a brief moment, in the minds of millions, grand – whether good or bad.

—

I have had periods when I felt very much like I was literally someone else. Once, driving down a highway at 140 km/h, I was convinced I was a young Bob Dylan speeding to go make a new record. Todd Haynes' anti-biopic *I'm Not There*, which fractured Dylan's portrayal by casting a myriad of actors in the role within the film, had just come out and it had taken a grip on my vulnerable mind. But, more to the point, removing accountability of the self during such episodes raises murky ongoing questions of ethics for those who encounter manic depression. Driving down the highway at dangerous high speeds, as some version of Bob Dylan, I had enough semblance of sanity that even I could see this. How does it feel?

—

Camera phones have changed the way we look at life and increased our access to out-of-the-ordinary moments. If we were reading about Russell's breakdown would it have the same visceral effect? There are videos of this kind that I will simply not watch. For example, I have read that there is a video of the actress and writer Carrie Fisher acting out her mania on a cruise ship because her medication was out of whack. I have watched a video of her on YouTube talking about the incident, but I refuse to go looking for the footage. To do so, I feel, would be to humiliate both myself and the recently dead Fisher, her memory and legacy as a mental health advocate.

—

These recent examples provide news media with two narratives to pursue. The first is to report on the example of extreme behaviour in an admonishing tone, and second, to return to the report with a revelation that the subject was suffering from a recently diagnosed case of mania. This doubles their readership and stretches their admonishment – first of the subject, and then, secondly, of their audience for not considering the possibility of a psychotic break when reading the first article. This is how news media thrives today.

This was true for Jason Russell. TMZ joked about the video in their initial release. News services followed up with family statements and the commentary turned to a more sombre mood. It can happen in real time too. On *The Young Turks* – an online commentary show on YouTube – a panel of journalists discussed the video of his breakdown, laughing throughout and joking about the situation: 'Oh boy ... Stop Russell 2012? If there were no drugs involved I feel worse for him.' The panellists then tried to temper their comments with stated sympathy for Russell.

—

When the point of crisis is isolated in news reporting like this, it appears as a strange, otherworldly moment – a ragged and ripped disjuncture in time where a human suddenly doesn't act human, or what we think of as human – and so, often you have to piece the rest of the story together yourself.

—

Mania is humiliating. It forces one into behaviours that are socially shunned and shamed. Wayne Koestenbaum's short book *Humiliation* has been a guide for my thinking. He writes: 'Imagine a society in which humiliation is essential – as a rite of passage, as a passport to decency and civilisation, as a necessary shedding of hubris.' Was this not true of Jason Russell, falling from grace? He was humiliated to bring him down to our level – disgusting, vulgar – and it saved him from becoming any more sanctimonious. We literally could not bear any more proselytising from him or any of his Invisible Children. Koestenbaum again: 'Humiliation has its rewards. Among them: the privilege of being seen as exemplary. The pleasure of being a spectacle. The perk of visibility, of becoming legible'. So, these rewards – 'the pleasure of being a spectacle' – are true of mania too.

—

Part of the reason I have come to write this book in short paragraphs is partly in homage to collage-like nonfiction – as a particular nod to Koestenbaum's methods and style in *Humiliation* – but it's also because this is how my mind works most of the time. It might be the medication or it might just be me. Experiencing ongoing problems with concentration is a terrible thing for an essayist or reader to contend with. It only seems surmountable if you rewire the format in which you write – so there's that. I only have the attention span to read parts of books, flitting between pages, but never locking down much of a linear thread. At the start of writing this book, I only had the attention span to watch trailers of films, not the films themselves, making the critical analysis required for these paragraphs very difficult indeed. My publisher has asked me to assure you that I got there in the end – coming out of the manic state that might have coloured early drafts of this book – and that I found my powers of concentration again.

—

To the best of my knowledge, there doesn't exist any video of me in a manic state. I mean, why would there be? I'm not famous. I don't hang around cameras all that much. What would the camera have captured if I had been famous, or louder? The worst I got was this: smashing glasses, knocking over a coffee table, screaming uncontrollably at others, breaking and entering a couple of times, hitting myself in the side of the head repeatedly with my own clenched fist, throwing a large painting at my dad, down the length of a hallway. It missed him, but the intention hit us both hard. It is best to put these things up front and get them out of the way. What if there had been video?

—

There are sites of mania, zones where an attack is more likely to take place. Some cities are seemingly designed with this in mind – the bright lights and noise of Las Vegas are conducive to manic spending – whereas others simply might provide a personal connection for the manic depressive. I, for instance, long for Californian air and vistas, but Los Angeles is dangerous for me: the rhythms of cities can be manic in and of themselves. Sometimes it's better that I sit in a quiet suburb and rage in solitude. I'd be safe and warm, if I was in LA, but that might also not be so true for me. No more parties in LA, Kanye West pleads, with good reason.

—

An Italian summer is certainly a site for mania. In Luca Guadagnino's film *A Bigger Splash* – a remake of the Italian-French film *La Piscine (The Swimming Pool)* and the novel of the same name – which is set on Pantelleria, a small volcanic isle off the Sicilian coast, Ralph Fiennes, from the first scene until his last, embodies mania and its organic connections with nudity as a hyper-projection of self-possession and an extreme visual marker of concrete confidence better than any other piece of culture I can think of. Fiennes plays Harry, the former lover of a rock star, played by a mute Tilda Swinton – whose muteness only amplifies Fiennes' rapid patter. Harry travels to the small Italian island seemingly to project himself on to everyone around him and try to reclaim his former love.

Fiennes' Harry wants everyone to tune in to the same frequency as his moods. In a central scene in the film, he pulls The Rolling Stones' *Emotional Rescue* from a collection of LPs and puts it on, enthusiastically promoting it to the small gathering in a light-filled lounge room. His dancing, as the song comes on, is of the 'so bad it's good' kind – flailing arms, jerky hips – delivered in a way that invites the others to join him, even if they can't keep up with his speed. It is a perfect physical expression of mania. This is about volume, in both its aural and quantitative meanings. Give them everything, and expect everything in return.

Once he has their attention though, Harry abandons them to go it alone. He walks outside – thrust along by Mick Jagger's pulsating falsetto – and continues dancing, under a burning sun, alone. Such is the pull of self-possession.

Later in the film, drunk on his own performance, Harry persuades an entire karaoke bar to join him in singing – badly, as bad as his dancing – Metropole's Italo-disco (or Disco Spaghetti) classic 'Miss Manhattan'. He entices Swinton's Marianne to join him, even though doing so would be damaging to her vocal cords. Does mania need collective recognition to be fuelled? There's no direct reference in the film that Fiennes' character has a history of manic depression – although there are telltale signs, such as excessive drug use and his general vibe of abandoned decorum. The *Guardian*'s film critic Peter Bradshaw suggested in his review of the film that Harry was 'bipolar without the down phase' alongside being 'a toxic narcissist and exhibitionist' and 'unable to stop talking'.

—

Is a naked man more of an affront to common cultural sensibilities than a naked woman? The Australian film critic Joanna Di Mattia considered Fiennes' nudity in a think piece for the literary magazine *Kill Your Darlings*, writing that 'Harry is a hurricane of sexual energy, relentlessly moving and thrusting about ... His clothing accentuates his carnality – he's prone to forgetting to button his shirts – and he's partial to promenading poolside without his pants.' Di Mattia distinguishes the film from the typical Hollywood production, which would normally shy away from male nudity: 'As a European arthouse film, *A Bigger Splash* affirms our expectations of how nudity can be approached in a system where full frontal male nudity is neither cause for alarm nor a source of humour. It simply *is*.' And, yet, it rarely *is*. The shock of Fiennes standing naked, often while others are clothed, is tangible. It points to his disregard for social conventions, but from where is that disregard born?

—

Fiennes sits naked, yet wrapped in a towel, after a drunken night swim. He is with Paul (played by Matthias Schoenaerts), his antagonist and romantic competition for the affections of Tilda Swinton's rock star Marianne, drinking from a stolen bottle of wine, which Paul cannot touch following a stint in rehab and a dramatic suicide attempt. He tells Paul he has been teaching himself some Italian, finally, and he rattles off some words and phrases:

> *Cacasentenze*: Someone who pretends to be very smart, who won't stop talking. 'One who shits sentences.' And

28

my favourite is *vomitare l'anima*: 'To puke your guts up.' Literally, 'to vomit your soul'.

Paul asks Marianne, earlier in the film, if Harry ever shuts up. He doesn't shut up, until he does. We see in flashbacks of Harry elements that suggest his excess of character being a kind of fixed personhood, but does the sharp sun of Pantelleria's island paradise serve to brighten him, to light him up and set him off? Part of the experience of mania is surely being on a permanent vacation – and anyone who has overstayed a holiday knows what that feels like. There is certainly a sense of overstaying your welcome when it comes to an elongated elevated mood such as mania. You're also always a guest: your stay *is* imposed on others. Stay at the party too long and you'll undoubtedly piss off the hosts.

—

What happens when the chief symptoms of a disease are so pleasure-related? There are times when I wish I were ill, as that side of the illness for me isn't associated at all with sickliness. In fact, illness for those who know mania is its exact opposite – a driving sense of strength and invincibility, and, along with this, a feeling of supreme healthiness. This contradiction causes all sorts of chaos. I miss my manias – a deeply dangerous, potentially deadly desire to go back. Fun can carry an element of danger – what happens when your pursuit of fun is pathological?

—

The moods we actively desire, that we pursue, are those entire industries – medical and otherwise – are built on aspiring to:

elation, euphoria, joy. If these feelings are experienced during a state of mania, afterwards the memory of them comes with the feeling that they were somehow manufactured, that your own feelings were, somehow, fraudulent. It is the same, one supposes, as saying that depression is not quite the same as sadness. An imbalance cannot be the exact thing. So there is something metallic, chalky and not quite right about remembering these feelings.

—

What of enthusiasm, obsession, and the regular, occasional forms of excess? So much of mania could, so easily, be mistaken for exuberance: 'A fun time had by all'. Kay Redfield Jamison's book *Exuberance: The Passion for Life* explores, in part, the connections between mania and emotions that relate to pleasure. It would take a psychologist diagnosed with manic depression, as Redfield Jamison is, to write such a treatise on unbridled joy – but why does mania have to intrude on this work? If mania is pure exuberance, it should be prodded – how does it come to be so? What is set off in the mind – in the delicate balance of brain chemistry – to send 'sufferers' (another term should be applied, such as 'experiencers') into such enthusiastic champagne bubbliness?

—

Sometimes it really just feels like an excess of personality – and that you have to burn through it in order to rid yourself of it. You could be two people, or provide enough personal energy to fuel two people. Your rapid speech fills in for another, but also doesn't let you get a word in.

—

For me, the most consistent pursuit of this 'fun', its defining feature, was a need to drive. This led to uncharacteristically criminal behaviour, or close enough. I came very near to stealing a car in Melbourne – luckily, I wasn't hardwired to hotwire. I didn't know how to get the thing started without a set of keys. I did smash its window with a chunk of concrete I had found somewhere, and then sitting inside for a while, searching for cash or keys.

—

It felt like an overcorrection from depression. A car careening that takes too swift a turn in the opposite direction. And then it goes off road.

—

Depression is harder to write about – it causes me to flinch. Who would want to go back and pick through the ashen remains of a house levelled by a painful fire? My memories of my manias are largely fond, and intoxicating. I want to go back to them, back to that place of fun and play. But I can't – or won't – go back to the manias. They are, ultimately, dangerous – and that dissonance, that play and fun can be dangerous, and should be avoided, is just something that I will have to live with.

—

Indeed, in my mind, the periods of mania are stronger as memories. The periods in which they existed were heightened by nature, so of course they stand out, but it is just how much pleasure was experienced at the time that make them so seductive to recall. I felt more fully myself – gifted with a level of self-confidence that few will ever obtain – but there is doubt that this was even ever me. If I look back on the destruction that this self-possession caused I want to be forgiven – 'It was not me, it was the disease' – but to achieve that absolution I need to, surely, forgo everything during that made me *me* at the time. I don't know. That's what I struggle with now. The most terrifying aspect of the disorder is that part of the experience relates to the sudden and total absence of anxiety. It is not quite like the lack of inhibitions brought about by alcohol consumption – though alcohol intake and abuse can certainly be one of its comorbid symptoms – though it is close. It doesn't make things blur, it makes them steely sharp, everything locks into place and your goals are in sight always. Solely ambitious people are typically pretty awful to be around. I had suddenly become one of them.

—

In his superlative work of ultra-hyper-pure-digressive non-fiction, *Out of Sheer Rage*, British-born author Geoff Dyer writes about an episode of depression he suffered while travelling in Rome. It wasn't his first time with the illness, and as is often the case with chronic conditions, he was beginning to understand the nature of the beast better:

> Now that dodge – getting out of depression by
> becoming interested in depression – only works once.
> There might be more to learn about it but I'm not
> interested. The only thing that interests me about
> depression is staying well clear of it.

This is not exactly a book about depression. When I do talk about it I focus on the upswing of coming out of depression: mania and hypomania. Not everyone who suffers through a bout of depression experiences this particular attendant condition, as it is typically reserved for those living with Bipolar Affective Disorder (I or II, take your pick really) or cyclothymia. And that is something you can dodge more than once, and, unfortunately, take great pleasure in.

—

Part of living with manic depression is reconciling two separate disorders: mania and depression. The complexity is impossible to describe. The psychoanalyst Darian Leader evokes Spike Milligan determining that the 'bad could not contaminate the good'. For Milligan it was 'absolute: the two traits had to be kept categorically apart'.

—

Someone, somewhere, says bluntly: 'Nobody needs another misery memoir.'

—

There are other absences in a book like this, of course – absences of the people on the other side, those who care and care for me. I can't tell everyone's story, and yet how strange that these absences are also the story.

—

I want to actively resist memoir, and the personal essay, but if I do, how am I going to give you a view of what it was like for me? How do I provide some sense of the interiority of this experience? So, I, like many writers before me, give in.

—

My second extended bout of mania occurred as my thirtieth birthday loomed, and remained in full swing for some time after that anniversary passed. This episode came fully wrapped in a bad year, in which I had resigned from a stressful, all-consuming job and lost a good friend to suicide. I had been severely depressed prior to this, walking around with a pain in my head. I would wake up in the morning and wish I was still asleep, and would spend most mornings willing myself back into a slumber. I had done the stupid thing of coming off my medication without consulting a doctor because I thought I was right again, and so I welcomed the New Year believing it was to be my last (that it turned out to be someone else's broke my heart a million times). Then, as sure as the approaching spring, the old enthusiasms returned with a vengeance. Not having the same work responsibilities and facing a personal milestone sent me into a strange daze. I wanted to 'go quite naked'. This was a more conscious decision than that which Jason Russell made – the difference between hypomania and acute psychosis is largely one of control.

—

Canberra has been the consistent site of my manias. Across all three major episodes I have experienced, I have ended up in Canberra. During the second episode I made a return. I hadn't been to Canberra in years, and knowing that I wanted to work on a book about naturism in Australia, I decided to try and find Kambah Pool, which was only a vague memory in my mind at the time. I drove out to the secluded spot, nestled in between rolling hills and an Arthur Boyd landscape lookalike backdrop. It had a picture-book quality to it along the drive and I had to pull over on the side of the road to take in the scene. In there, somewhere, there is a connection to my identity at the time – a desire to be vulgar. I decided I would travel to all of Australia's nude beaches as research for my book. I only made it to two. I asked my friend Weeds, a photographer, to come with me. I was writing for *Archer* magazine – a new magazine dedicated to ideas around sexuality, gender and identity – and I had planned to visit some of the nude beaches my grandmother used to drag me to as a child. My mood at the time was more about creative energy unspent than anything else.

Before we hit Canberra though, Weeds and I were in the actual weeds. We were looking for a nudist beach just outside of Melbourne but we couldn't find the right one – or we had found it, but we weren't sure where you were actually allowed to denude, because there was no one else around. We walked for nearly an hour trying to find the spot, but there were no markers to signal where it was okay to strip your clothes off. By the time we got to the end of the long, lonely stretch, we were suddenly in the middle of a throng of wetsuit-clad surfers, running out into the whitewash to paddle to a break. We were confused, and then realised we had passed the exact spot half an hour back.

From there, Weeds and I drove out of Melbourne in a rented car, in which I had already driven down from Sydney a few days before (driving is always there; to my loved ones, if I am seen at a rental car company, call my psychiatrist). We were supposed to be driving out to a three-hatted restaurant, in rural Victoria to photograph and interview the head chef, but we were running late, and the general manager of the restaurant was on the phone screaming at me because of this, and I hadn't actually placed the piece with any publication, so it was all built on a lie (typical of mania, I was moving faster than the pace of normal business hours: creatively, the foundations of what I was attempting were falling apart as I built on top of them).

So we diverted and dog-legged onto the Hume, arriving in Canberra with one goal: to make our way to Kambah Pool – a spot my grandmother had taken me to on a family holiday when I was eleven. After a night in a cheap hotel, Weeds and I drove out there. I had already been to the pool a few times in my hypomanic daze.

That year I had been invited to take part in Junket – a three-day self-described un-conference run by the youth media website Junkee – in which hundreds of distinguished young roughly millennial 'thought leaders' came together to discuss different aspects of contemporary society in what was intended to be a pretty practical way. The curator of participants sent long emails outlining the ambition of the conference:

> The aim of Junket is to share ideas, get advice, be
> inspired, innovate, teach, learn, network and have fun
> – all with the (suitably ambitious) aim of helping set the
> agenda for Australia's future.

No small feat to set the agenda for Australia's future. This of course, was in keeping with the political, countercultural undercurrent programmed into the design of the conference.

I was fielding calls from Canberra friends who were concerned no one local had been invited. They were going to bust down the hotel's doors and I was thinking of giving them my room number and place at the table. I had driven down in a rental car I couldn't afford – despite being sponsored by a major airline company, no travel costs would be covered – and wore myself out alone at the wheel. The Federal Highway has oppressive visual qualities expressed via a flat blandness – the road goes on for what feels like forever, bearing down on you with its infinite expanse. Mania has the potential to increase sensitivity to both visual and auditory senses – there were times that even the smallest sound alone could send me into a violent rage – and so even something as boring as the Hume becomes too loud. My eyes blurred and gave out. I was tired to the point of hysteria, and at rest stops would walk around in circles while hyperventilating. I had with me a camera, which I couldn't afford – I spent my last pay cheque on it, in the hope that I could become a wedding or food photographer for rent money, but had no real idea of how to get into the business. I only used the camera through these months of hypomania.

—

Weeds and I walk to the NGA from our hotel room. There, I found a small, modest painting by Frank Crozier titled *Deadbeat* painted in 1918. A soldier in khaki sits alone, under a clouded, complicated sky, his rifle leaning on his pack, his legs pulled up to his body and he just stares. In my mind, I am hearing: 'This is a TV show. There's never been a TV show about a returning soldier with post-traumatic stress disorder (PTSD) and *Deadbeat* – more contemporary feeling than its

1918 prescription by Crozier – is the perfect title for it. Six episodes. I'll write and produce it. Just write it now, and it will be good.' This is the problem with mania – the speed at which the idea came to me, and the time in which it came, now makes me question it entirely. I mean, it's not that bad an idea. In fact, it probably is a good idea. There *hasn't* been a show about a soldier grappling with issues relating to mental ill health in this country, and it seems like a worthy subject to tackle in a longform television program. But I am not the person to write it. I've never written for television, and don't really think about the format nor the form. I contact a friend who has written a television show, seeing if he would be interested in collaborating, and he agrees it is a good idea – but, still, it remains ready to rot because it's associated with the state of my mind at the time it came to me.

———

During this time, nature thrummed in front of me – everything I saw seemed heightened somehow, as if someone had turned the colour up on plant life, or my eyes had been retuned to see more sharply. I couldn't stop taking photographs of flowers on my camera phone. I would genuflect on hot asphalt in front of pedestrian blooms to get the right shot. So, it was little wonder that I was ecstatic in silty river water, overseen by spindly trees in a bush setting. It was as close to religious ecstasy as I'll ever get; God, if one existed, could not invent a way of touching your soul in such a deeply felt way. I was sitting naked on a rock, when a fly tried to creep into my foreskin – surely a sign from a higher power. In the photographs, which Weeds sent me, I am nude, except I am wearing a pair of sunglasses. I eventually submitted a mock-up of the book to the Australia Council for the Arts in the hopes of receiving funds to produce and distribute the book myself. This was my insanity. I'm glad they didn't give me any money; I would have spent it too fast, on things unrelated to the project – very likely a flight to Los Angeles. Only trouble there. *No more parties in LA.*

—

That manic episode stretched from late September 2015 until somewhere in January 2016. That could be deduced from the number of pictures I took alone. It's not my most recent episode – that would take place at the start of 2017, and was the most dangerous manic episode I've had yet. This isn't just my story. Part of my critical thinking about the cultural identity of manic-depression has always been formed through others as much as myself. Along the way I have reckoned with figures in recent history who have had varying degrees of success in telling their own stories, and I've learnt from them. In some cases, people – writers, mostly – have owned and told their own stories to a point that it has changed the way people talk and think about manic depression.

—

Now, sitting in front of a blank document, I am naked but not yet nude, afraid of what is to come, what is not yet said.

WAYS
OF
READING

2
BLACK BACKPACK, CROWBAR, TORCH, BOOK

During the height of it – and in a work such as this we need to register some sort of height – there were lost books. Here is one example of how: I packed a black backpack with a crowbar, a battery-powered torchlight and a copy of *Broken Open*, a book by Craig Hamilton, a local sports reporter, about his psychotic breakdown during the Sydney 2000 Olympics. The memoir, which I was yet to open, had been given to me by my very intuitive grandmother. I had dreamt of walking around inside a house, a specific house, a few doors down from my own. The house – a modernist beachfront property, whose rough, beige stucco rendering appropriately mimicked sand – had occupied my mind for months. I had been watching the house – which seemed to me, at the time, to be only ever used as a holiday residence – on long beach walks as I recovered from a depressive episode that winter. I imagined that once I was inside, sitting in front of the large black paintings on those sleek big-bottomed leather couches that I would finally be able to begin to feel well again, and that the house would be mine. I don't know what I was thinking – you can't steal a house just by sitting in it, unless you can claim squatter's rights. Going outside into the ocean-cooled air, and slipping

into the sleek black of the night, I first circled the house looking for the easiest way in. Finding none, I wormed my way
into the crawl space beneath the house and considered using
the crowbar to break up through the floorboards. I did not
want to smash glass (too loud) but splintering through wood
seemed an okay option for some reason. I would be coming at
things from a different angle. Then I laughed off this option
as surely impossible and crawled back out to walk up onto
the deck and found that a window had been left slightly
ajar. I went and tried to prise it open a little wider, and as I
began to tear at the flyscreen material through the window
– a scratchy sound like Velcro separating – a voice came at
me from inside the room; a sort of dog's growl, playing with
the words 'What' and 'are' and 'you' and 'doing'. The order
of the words didn't seem right to me. Whoever was saying
them sounded like they were not sure what they were saying
and knew that I was not sure what I was hearing. The exact
meaning would only register later. For the moment there was
a sudden rush of adrenalin that nearly crippled me from its
pulsating surge, ripping through chest and limbs. I dropped
everything except the crowbar, which I clutched tightly to
my chest as I ran down the steep garden front and on to the
beach. I tore through lantana and birds of paradise and hit the
dunes hard. I ran around and hid down the side of another,
more modest beach house, a house that hadn't even crossed
my mind to break into. From down low, I could see that all
of the lights of the house on the hill were being turned on.
There was a figure pacing, clearly on the telephone. I waited
for police sirens, and some time later, when there were none,
I began to take the long way around to my house. I realised
soon enough that I had left the copy of *Broken Open* behind

and that my grandmother's name was signed in the top corner of the title page, with that distinctive surname of ours, which would be enough for anyone to track her down. I never heard a word from anyone about it. I never dared to ask. Three or four nights later I would be in a psychiatric ward anyway, sleeping under the heavy sedation of tranquillisers, a concrete diagnosis imminent.

3

A SHORT TOUR THROUGH THE CULTURAL HISTORY OF MANIC DEPRESSION

The modern definition of manic depression, indeed its earliest push towards that order of phrasing, was logged in a little act of madness. The French psychiatrist Jules Baillarger delivered a lecture in early 1854 on his concept of *folie à double forme* (alternating insanity, or more literally: madness double form), in which he detailed that a patient may experience both mania and depression. Almost immediately Baillarger's colleague Jean-Pierre Falret came out to say that he had already documented such a condition in his theory of *folie circulaire* (circular insanity). Baillarger then accused Falret of outright plagiarism. Falret kept quiet on the matter, while Baillarger continued to prosecute his case for the rest of his life. In either case, *folie circulaire* or *folie à double forme* became the prominent definition of manic depression until the German psychiatrist Emil Kraepelin began using the exact term and, eventually, published his foundational and frequently updated *Manic-depressive Insanity and Paranoia*.

The idea of these two competing theories, complete with sparring French psychiatrists, feels like it could be the plot of some weirdo European comic novel. But the history of psychiatry, psychotherapy and psychoanalysis has always been a little *nuts* in and of itself. When I first saw a psychologist during a long depressive period, preceding my first experience of mania, I went into her office knowing full well that she was feuding with another psychologist, a colleague at the same clinic. I can't remember how I knew this beyond rumour but it gave me a quick induction in developing a healthy scepticism towards those who treat you. That could be passed on to those who write about manic depression who do not suffer from it. The history of the psychiatrically ill has been one of a dispossession of voice. The stories of those who have suffered from conditions such as manic depression have largely been recorded in medical reporting. The unexpected outcome of the definition of a fixed diagnosis was to provide a name for a set of extreme symptoms that people could, increasingly, identify with. The ability to speak from this position increased as stigma relating to a diagnosis was challenged throughout the twentieth century, leading us into the twenty-first.

Neither Falret nor Baillarger, however, went on to be mentioned much throughout popular histories of manic depression. The figure that very much took their place was Kraepelin, who superseded those who preceded him with *Manic-depressive Insanity and Paranoia* – creating the name that would stick through the act of distinguishing the disorder from schizophrenia and melancholia. His treatise came at the turn of the century, setting the nomenclature for a disorder whose visibility would rise in years to come (part of this had to do with the novelty of the terms he used, especially *depressive*, which wasn't in common use). *Manic-depressive Insanity and Paranoia* didn't quite take hold, however, until it was translated into English in 1921. Kraepelin was working against modes of psychoanalysis and the Freudian schools of the time, as he was conducting his research in an almost purely medical mode, using classic diagnostic methods. He collected cases and used symptoms as data; according to the psychiatrist and author David Healy in his *Mania: A Short History of Bipolar Disorder*, the *DSM-III* was 'supposedly an expression of a neo-Kraepelinian movement, which sought to return psychiatry to its clinical roots in detailed observation of patients, after an interlude in which the discipline dallied with psychoanalysis'. Indeed, Kraepelin's 'disease model' of studying manic depression, as compared to taking a psychoanalytical view, has largely held true over time, as the dominant mode of diagnosis, treatment and its cultural starting point.

Kraepelin was also a globalist – he travelled as far as Indonesia for his research – and apparently, according to Healy, he was something of a bore. Yet he is an important figure. Beginning with Kraepelin's definitions and descriptions at the turn of the twentieth century, manic depression came increasingly into view. The culture explored it carefully, but kept its realities hidden away, often in asylums. It would take a brave few to explode it open and let the rest of us in.

⎯

The effectiveness of lithium for treating mania, acting as a mood stabiliser, was discovered in Australia in the late 1940s. The psychiatrist John Cade had grown up in the shadow of mental asylums. Cade's father, also a doctor, had served in Gallipoli and France during the First World War, and returned experiencing 'war-weariness'. He later took positions in mental institutions throughout Victoria. Cade Jnr, as a result, moved into medicine, almost naturally. Growing up alongside the patients of the mental institutions for which his father worked surely had a significant influence on the young man. Lithium turned out to be the first effective medication, helping to scale back electroconvulsive therapy (ECT) and lobotomies as the primary treatments for mania. Cade cooked up his experiments with lithium in an unused kitchen at the Bundoora Repatriation Mental Hospital in Melbourne, a site for treating 'shell shock'.

There is an uncredited photograph of John Cade, searchable on Getty Images, wearing thick black specs and holding out a small white pill between his index finger and thumb. He can't help but look like a pusher in the picture, but the revolution that Cade's little pill has had on the treatment of mania cannot be understated. I, however, have never taken lithium, having been prescribed newer drugs, but I have friends who swear by it still. I take a combination of medications now. The concept of the drug cocktail is well known to manic-depressives. One drug I've been on for nearly ten years, a familiar friend who has been around as long as the diagnosis. It is primarily known as an anticonvulsant prescribed for epileptics. No one seems to completely understand why it also works as a mood stabiliser for manic depressives. Like lithium, it comes with its own mysteries. The other is a straight up sedative. A tiny pink pill, it approaches me like a bruiser with bulging arms in a bar and knocks me the fuck out. Life is filled with unknowns, but not knowing quite why or how a certain new medication works is somewhat terrifying – taking it, not knowing how it affects you bodily, what its long-term effects might be, causes unease. It is one of the reasons people taper off their medication, but what lies beyond that pharmaceutical renunciation can be scarier still.

—

In the Chinese-Korean slacker film, *A Quiet Dream*, a melancholic North Korean defector, played sensitively by Park Jung-bum, takes his bipolar medication while hanging out with his drop-kick friends at a tent bar in the backyard of their collective crush. His bipolarity is a punchline for his friends, but his sweet, soft-spoken nature, and the fact that he took his medication out in the open, made me cheer him on.

—

Sitting in a New York café in mid-2015, I opened the *New York Times* weekend supplement to find a cover story by Jaime Lowe, writing about visiting the world's largest salt flat, Salar de Uyuni in Bolivia. Lowe tables her own experiences with manic depression and treatment with lithium. Trekking the flats, Lowe looks out onto the salt, and observes that 'The lithium we have on Earth now – part stardust, part primordial dust and part earth dust – is a constituent part of our planet, one that sometimes shapes personalities.' I kept that copy of the *New York Times* magazine, bringing it home with me, and it now sits on my coffee table – a prized possession. The writing of others lights the way.

The Brooklyn-based Taylor Beck wrote in an opinion piece, 'Kin by mania: The bond I feel with other bipolar people is inexplicable':

> The more of us I meet, the less I feel like a mutant. In the way my friends think, talk, and act, I see myself. They are not bored. Not complacent. They engage. Theirs is a family I'm proud to be part of: curious, driven, chasing hard, caring intensely.

I shared the article with many of my bipolar blood brothers and sisters, and, collectively, we nodded in agreement. We were less mutants in the reading of Beck's words.

—

David Healy is a professor of psychiatry with a healthy, if occasionally overzealous, scepticism towards pharmaceutical approaches to treating manic depression. He isn't afraid to seem dismissive, and he had harsh words for the terminology around manic depression:

> As of 2000, the word manic-depressive had all but vanished from the American clinical map. This vanishing began in the mid-1990s. When Fred Goodwin and Kay Jamison published the largest monograph on the disorder in 1990, it was entitled *Manic-Depressive Illness*. Jamison's 1993 and 1995 books also refered to manic-depressive illness rather than bipolar disorder. It took the development and marketing of mood stabilisers for everyone to become bipolar. This process began in 1995, when Abbott Laboratories received a license for valproate for the treatment of mania.

The incursions of the cure on nomenclature can be attributed to these marketing exercises. This is the power of words debated by PR people to help sell a disease, and its medications, to the masses. 'Manic-depressive', one imagines, was voted down in some cold, clinical boardroom, due to its stigma, public history and general air of menace. Bipolar, flat and accessible (sellable), became the cause. Redfield Jamison rejected the term in *An Unquiet Mind,* and others have rebelled, choosing to nominate manic depression as their preferred term. If my omission of the term so far hasn't made this clear, I don't like the term 'bipolar'. In fact, I actively distrust it. 'Bipolar' points towards a palatability and a mass appeal that may serve to destigmatise the disorder, but in the end goes some way to erasing its core elements. The poles are not quite equal – in intensity or otherwise – and bipolar suggests a kind of gentle see-sawing between the two, an expedition from which you can come back. I use it on occasion when referring to clinical diagnoses – but I still cry bullshit.

—

While Kraepelin didn't mention Falret nor Baillarger in his findings, there is something useful in a broader metaphoric sense to the term *folie circulaire* – which translates to 'circular insanity' – and points to the rapid thought cycles, often looping back on themselves, in a mixed manic state. *Folie à double forme* simply has a nice ring to it.

If Kraepelin and co created a set of criteria, they might have done so in order that others could confess to identifying with these criteria. Throughout the twentieth century – and into the twenty-first – the symptoms and suffering of mental ill health have made for rousing literature. The confessional form – largely memoir, occasionally the personal essay – in which writers have disclosed their struggles with mental instability has surely provided relief for any number of authors, while serving readers with a certain fix. The medical literature might not be widely accessed, but popular fiction and general nonfiction have assisted in gesturing towards its findings.

—

How did the medical language of these developments seep into mainstream culture over the century, and form a unique cultural identity for those living with manic depression? Through the statistics, it becomes clear that it is a disease – more than any other – that is owned by literature. And it owns writers more than any other disorder. The statistics, like most statistics, are scary. Alice W Flaherty states in *The Midnight Disease* (2005) that writers are ten times more likely to be manic depressive than the rest of the population, and poets are a staggering forty times more likely. The overriding concern then becomes a variation on the classic chicken-or-egg question: does the act of writing invite mental illness, or does writing come from some need to cope with it? It's not as clear-cut as one or the other, but if it were solely the former, who would go into it willingly? And if so, what can we do to make writers more aware of the risks? Do you put up a white warning sticker, like on packets of cigarettes, so that every time you bought a Moleskine notebook or a Uni-ball pen, they would be emblazoned with 'Writing May Cause Harm'?

—

The connections between writing and mental illness were clear to me when I began trying to write professionally for the first time. When I wrote prose, the same thing always tripped me up: trying to succeed beyond realistic expectations. The desire to be above the level I was at could stop me from progressing on a draft entirely. I would be halted mid-sentence, with little else to do but stew on why I'd stopped. In the slowed-down process of revising work with editors, depressive moods prevailed. I couldn't bring myself to email them on some days and would get up each morning frightened that the deadline – the hard finality of the word pressing down on me – was one day closer, or worse, one day behind me, unmet. I would finish multiple drafts, but the piece could never be good enough, never up to the exacting standards that I, like many young writers, had invented for myself. I would stare blankly at the computer, the Word doc refusing to edit itself. Individual sentences would make sense, but the whole would be irreversibly tangled. The reality of writing at a professional level is that the process isn't exactly cheery. It can, in fact, mimic manic depressive cycles: the inspiration that comes with an idea takes hold for weeks, bringing with it sleeplessness and excited energy, before slowly succumbing to the turgidity of rewriting and overworking.

—

F Scott Fitzgerald published *The Crack-Up* in three parts across the February, March and April issues of *Esquire* magazine in 1936. The series of short personal essays revealed Fitzgerald's struggles with a nervous disposition. *The Crack-Up* was released in book form in 1945, five years after Fitzgerald's death. The book was edited to include other pieces by Fitzgerald and was compiled by the literary critic Edmund Wilson. The reviews were not kind. Writing in the *New York Times*, William Du Bois called them 'unhappy pages' and 'more pathetic than moving'. Over time, the three essays which form the core of *The Crack-Up* would come to be considered classics, and would influence another generation of writers to admit to their fallibilities and explore their own mental anguish.

More than fifty years after *The Crack-Up*, for instance, the well-known American novelist and essayist William

Styron is credited with bringing this kind of memoir into the mainstream with *Darkness Visible*, a short book published in 1990, which grew out of a long essay published in *Vanity Fair* in 1989. Styron's book came with the subtitle 'A Memoir of Madness' but the work is largely confined to unipolar depression.

Styron explored his depressive episode with a kind of naïve curiosity – a writer carefully exploring new ground. Unipolar depression is no less serious than manic depression, yet for Styron it appeared as a one-off experience – a late-life aberration – and there is a risk in thinking that manic depression trumps depression in terms of stakes. When I went through the worst of it, many friends who had experienced depression reached out and told me, 'I know what you're going through', in response to which I couldn't help but think, 'Not really, you don't know it … not like this.' I can see that such 'us and them' thinking is potentially disastrous. The dialogue around both disorders is forever entwined, and the breakthroughs in research in one can often help the other. Indeed, writing about one form of mental ill health can have positive impacts for writing about other disorders. Styron, for instance, opened one door, without knowing that he would be letting someone else open the second.

—

In my mind, this 'someone else' is a writer, who has made full use of the lifelong nature of manic depression to build a powerful career around getting as close as possible to the effects of the disorder. She appears again and again in the literature; across my reading while I researched this book, she was easily the most quoted figure in other books about manic depression. In 1990, the American psychologist Kay Redfield Jamison co-authored the biomedical textbook *Manic Depressive Illness* with the psychiatrist Frederick Goodwin. In 1995, she then published *An Unquiet Mind*. This book differed in that it was a memoir, written from a very close first person point of view. It became clear, on reading, how the earlier book was written with such an empathic understanding for the condition it laid out.

Kay Redfield Jamison has a quiet, mild manner in her recorded public appearances, challenging the usual conception of a manic depressive. She is softly spoken, gentle and measured in her speech. Part of the overall effect of Redfield Jamison's presence within the public sphere is to normalise and destigmatise the disorder. Her professional achievements are the primary testament to that, although one must be careful not to ignore those who struggle with professional stability due to the disorder. Reading *An Unquiet Mind* one is also struck by the even-handed prose, which borders on being flat. It would be too easy – and unfair – to describe the writing as clinical; Redfield Jamison had been influenced by her own previous writing in producing academic works, reports and medical textbooks. This working life was at risk due to the new book. Redfield Jamison had a difficult decision to 'come out' as manic depressive, with all its professional consequences. The book is in large part a portrait of gradual disclosures to a series of colleagues and, most movingly, lovers. That this culminates in the publication of the book as a final and firm admission is part of Redfield Jamison's power.

—

The cure is often seen as a curse for the writer. This is a dangerous position to take. Many writers have railed against medication and voiced concern about its effects on their creativity and productivity. This cycle is driven by a kind of vanity. David Foster Wallace famously went off his medication – Nardil – after experiencing severe stomach pains following a meal at a Persian restaurant, which may have reacted badly with the drug. According to his biographer, DT Max, Foster Wallace 'was becoming more convinced that Nardil might be getting in the way of *The Pale King*'. He was tapered off the medication with the help of his doctor – the safest way to stop taking medication, if necessary, is to have the supervision of a medical professional – but the decision would prove fatal. *The Pale King* would ultimately remain unfinished following Foster Wallace's suicide in 2008, though it was published posthumously in 2011. Many creative people misguidedly believe that medication is tampering with their focus and drive.

—

Concern for the wellbeing of the writer runs through the history of manic depression. The effects of medication and treatment rise to the top of most writing on the subject. Redfield Jamison spends much of *An Unquiet Mind* detailing her internal debates about going on lithium. I identified most closely with her when reading her description of how her ability to 'read, comprehend and remember' became compromised as a direct result of her lithium dosage:

> Reading, which had been at the heart of my intellectual
> and emotional existence, was suddenly beyond my
> grasp. I was used to reading three or four books a week;

now it was impossible. I did not read a serious work
of literature or nonfiction, cover to cover, for more
than ten years. The frustration and pain of this were
immeasurable. I threw books against the wall in a blind
fury and sailed medical journals across my office in a
rage.

I have taken medication that has adversely affected my concentration, along with medication which has caused blurred
vision. In a state of acute mania itself, it is unlikely that you
are going to find time – or the discipline – necessary to sit and
read. After I published a piece about my inability to finish
reading books, someone told me that she thought it was an
'extremely brave thing' to confess to. To be fair, I had not at
the time linked it to my experiences of mania, but for all the
links between creativity and manic depression – as outlined
by Redfield Jamison herself – there are an equal number of
destructive qualities, or simply banal blockages like a deferred
ability to read, and along with it all the connections to wider
culture and self-improvement reading provides. Then again,
I was too busy being a jerk to worry about any of that.

This was certainly bad news for a writer. Some of the
medications I took had side effects, which, as stated, included
an inability to concentrate. Others were rumoured to chew
away at your brain mass. I have a friend who describes herself as being monogamous to her books; that she only reads
the one thing at the one time. I am promiscuous. I am often
reading three or more books at once. I am greedy and sloppy
and an inattentive lover, who fails to get to the book's climax.
The books on my desk spill out and trip over each other, until
I get fed up with them, and place them in a towering pile,

beneath the desk where I cannot see them or have to deal with them in any way. I blame this on the Book Depository and its recommendation algorithm, for the fact that when I am only one hundred pages into a book, there is already another waiting for me to retrieve it from the letterbox, ready to be ripped open. But this is disingenuous – the blame lies at my own sloth-like feet.

Being a writer who is not particularly good at reading is a constant humiliation. This reminds me of the *Onion* parody of a weekend supplement, featuring a verbose David Foster Wallace on the cover with the confession 'I Never Learned To Read'. I so very much wanted that confession to be true when I first read it; for it not to be a parody, but a searing exposé. It would have made me feel much better about my own inability to finish books. But Geoff Dyer saved me by writing the essay 'Readers Block', explaining that we naturally go through periods where our attentiveness falters and we fall into a non-reading lull, especially as we get older. This makes the blow less forceful when I admit that I could not finish a certain book.

This is a bad confession to be making in a book of researched nonfiction. Please trust me that my messy, scatter-shot reading, in fact, makes for perfect nonfiction research.

—

Kay Redfield Jamison has consistently explored this connection between creativity and manic depression. She followed up her textbook with *Touched With Fire: Manic-Depressive Illness and the Artistic Temperament* in 1993. The book remains in print today and is easy enough to find. It bored me when I first read it. Redfield Jamison also briefly mentions writing poetry in her memoir, although she doesn't give many examples. So what do we expect from the manic depressive writer? Something more stylised? Something less studious? I see zigzags across the page in my mind. Clean copy, on first inspection, might not be desirable. This might be asking too much, and Redfield Jamison's cultural legacy is larger than her individual style.

In a brutal appendix attached to *Touched With Fire*, Redfield Jamison lists 'Writers, Artists, and Composers with Probable Cyclothymia, Major Depression, or Manic-Depressive Illness' to which she adds a key with which each name is marked: Asylum or psychiatric hospital, Suicide, or Suicide attempt. Some names contain two keys, none are marked thrice.

In publishing *Touched With Fire*, Redfield Jamison contributed greatly to a new form of literary biography. Her work was contemporaneous with Thomas C Caramagno's 1992 book *The Flight of the Mind*, which concerned itself with crafting an out-of-the-box biography of Virginia Woolf, focusing on her diagnosis of manic depression. The retroactive exploration of the mental health of literary figures would become a genre in itself, aided and abetted by Redfield Jamison's work on creativity and madness; Redfield Jamison contributed an afterword to *The Flight of the Mind*.

—

This extra-literary biographical approach was met with some scepticism when first published. In an occasionally reactionary essay written for the *London Review of Books* – covering both *Touched With Fire* and *An Unquiet Mind* – the novelist, essayist and memoirist Jenny Diski wrote about the approach

Redfield Jamison takes in her two books. Diski, who had written openly about her experiences during her lifetime with depression and early psychiatric hospitaliation, took issue with Redfield Jamison's *Touched With Fire*, and, in particular, her exploration of the lives of William Blake and other artists. Diski wrote, pointedly, 'The diagnosis is of no use to Blake, because he is dead. Is it of some help to his readers?'

Well, perhaps not general readers, but there is comfort for those who experience manic depression to find a line and legacy in those who have come before. Redfield Jamison's books can easily become talismans, recommended and shared freely, in their potential to make one feel far less alone and connected to others. Diski's scepticism is useful and her point is to not over-invest in such hypothetical diagnoses. And, she seems to ask, what would we do with these retroactive diagnoses? Diski says it is not a pertinent question, but asks anyway, 'Would Blake on lithium have been Blake?'

Diski simply seemed uneasy with Redfield Jamison's continuous connection between sufferers of manic depression and creativity:

> I do wonder what dismal effect books like *Touched with Fire* have on those sufferers of manic depression who do not find themselves compensated with artistic greatness, but only scuppered by a dreadfully debilitating illness.

'Dismal effect' appears harsh but Diski genuinely seems to be making this judgment through empathy for everyone who experiences psychological disorders. And there is an imbalance even here. Not everyone, after all, has access to the support networks – emotional, educational, financial or otherwise – to tell their own story, or to connect with those of others.

—

Diski's review was cheekily titled 'Having Half the Fun' and writing of a patient who showed signs of euphoria, Diski commented, 'This is the kind of mild mania that makes unipolars mutter grimly that bipolars have all the fun.'

—

The importance of a figure like Redfield Jamison is in the leadership she provides to a fractured group of identified sufferers. It is part of the reason she is so warmly received and why many look up to her. The truth is that those who live with manic depression aren't well served by a sense of community – the disease itself pushes away from this idea, and, much to its detriment, prefers individualism by nature – and this has had a flow-on effect to how sufferers are represented in political spheres. There isn't much in the way of a collective activist voice as there is in other parts of the disability sector. The question of whether manic depression and similar conditions qualify as a disability remains open. The fight now is to try and create more of a sense of community and sharing. That's not easy though. It's like the old joke about the anarchists' meeting: that no one showed up because no one could agree that time exists, let alone choose a time to hold the meeting.

—

Redfield Jamison's influence has in itself, inspired some mis-guided art. Paul Dalio, a protégé of the director Spike Lee, wrote a screenplay called *Mania Days*, which Lee showed an interest in producing. The film was eventually released and retitled as *Touched With Fire*, taking its name from Redfield Jamison's book. *The Washington Post* made the point that Dalio, unlike the directors of recent bipolar biopics, had been diagnosed with the condition himself. Dalio did some press with Redfield Jamison, as if wheeling her out legitimised the film, but in interviews Dalio seemed to take the wrong lessons from her book, and Redfield Jamison sat back during a long interview with Charlie Rose, saying little.

Touched With Fire is a film brimming with bad ideas executed poorly. Watching it in bed one hot day, I felt bewil-dered, viewing it through my fingers like a horror movie. I kept turning it off and hoping it wasn't real. This was the logical extreme of taking the diagnosis and turning it into a full cultural identity – to trade, in a cheap metallic way, in its cult iconography (the main character paints a room in Van Gogh's swirling nightscapes) and to take Redfield Jamison's theoretical inquiries and render them as bad cinema. If Dalio takes the human experience of mania and makes bad art out of it, it is hard to blame him – mania is intoxicating, and its individual biographical details appear to have great dramatic narrative potential. Individual personal narratives are impor-tant, as they go some way towards creating a collective cul-tural identity for the manic depressive. But that doesn't mean that you have to identify with, nor praise, each entry into the canon of crazy.

—

The overriding desire to narrativise one's life might come from the creative urge of the illness, certainly, but it might also result from the rote reproductions necessary in each medical encounter related to its treatment. I have probably had three major episodes: one in 2008, in which I was twisted out of shape to the point of being unrecognisable and which ended in my first hospitalisation, then one in 2015, in which all the pleasures in life came back to me in full force but which burned out at its own rate. My third mania just felt like going through the motions again. The first two both followed depressive episodes; the feeling was comparable to having a sense of taste return after losing it, but this return was so intense it made me indulge and gorge on everything. What does it mean to come of age with a mind always teetering on the edge of instability? I wanted to hold onto the diagnosis for dear life through the worst of it. The identity helped me weather the reality of the illness – what it was enacting, the damage it was causing around me. But again there was doubt. How much of my behaviour was just fumbling in early adulthood, hot over-enthusiasms of the age and just plain getting things wrong?

—

Do we feel special? Oliver Sacks, writing in the *New York Review of Books*, said that mania has 'special qualities'. These, according to Sacks, 'have been recognized and distinguished from other forms of madness since the great physicians of antiquity wrote on the subject'. Sacks qualifies this by going on to say, 'medical accounts, accounts from the outside, can never do justice to what is actually experienced in the course of such psychoses; there is no substitute here for firsthand accounts'. Memoirs have their place. Sacks singles out John Custance's *Wisdom, Madness and Folly: The Philosophy of a Lunatic* as a particular favourite of his. There is something deeply sincere about the position from which Custance writes – much of the book was composed from within an asylum, and in the aftermath of acute mania. His approach, then, is a methodological accounting of his manias and depressions, and the treatise is clearly an attempt to benefit future studies.

—

Custance's book, first published in 1952, has been out of print for decades. I had to order a copy from a secondhand bookseller in Dunedin and waited anxiously until it arrived. Sitting with it for a few days, it felt like the closest thing to what I was trying to achieve when writing about mania – to use oneself willingly as a sample to better understand the condition. Think of it as akin to donating organs (except you're alive). Custance offers much. He gives an exact timeline of his manias and depressions, and how they might coincide. He offers long appendixes about his exact experiences in hospitals and with treatment, hoping to improve conditions. He offers a sample of writing composed during an acute manic episode. He writes out a long set of rapid thought associations as he looks out the window of his ward, starting with the flock of seagulls he sees fly by, kicking off some word play between a sea gull and the homonym 'sea girl':

> Mermaids, i.e. 'Sea girls', sirens, Lorelei, Mother
> Seager's syrup, syrup of figs, the blasted fig-tree in the
> Gospels, Professor Joad who could not accept Jesus
> as the supremely perfect Man owing to particular

incident. Here the chain stops as I cannot remember the exact title of Joad's book, which was a confession of the failure of his agnosticism.

Custance's wit is dry throughout. There are stretches where he gets bogged down in esoteric theological musing and Jungian contemplation, but he also understands and communicates the duality of the disease better than anyone else I have read, and much of the book is structured around the idea of these dualities. Twinned chapters are called 'Universe of Bliss' and 'Universe of Horror', devoted to mania and depression respectively. In a chapter titled 'Fantasia of Opposites', Custance writes that 'manic-depression is a condition with two aspects in some sort of fundamental opposition to one another'. He describes these as forces of 'attraction' (mania) and 'repulsion' (depression) and makes clear that he chooses such words because they have both physiological and psychological meanings. Much of the book is concerned with whether manic depression has some physical element. Custance's senses are heightened during his manic episodes – in particular, he has extreme visual hallucinations (a psychotic symptom I have thankfully dodged) – and his account is in part a plea for his condition to be explored medically and seriously. This concern is echoed in Redfield Jamison's distaste for 'clinicians who somehow draw a distinction between the suffering and treatability of "medical illness" such as Hodgkin's disease or breast cancer, and psychiatric illness such as depression, manic depression, or schizophrenia'. Part of living with manic depression means fighting for its legitimacy, in both medical and cultural terms. It remains contested ground.

—

Custance's descriptions of the characteristics of his manic state don't quite line up with the contemporary *DSM* list, but are poetic and thoughtful, and are worth quoting in full:

> (I) Intense sense of well-being, (2) heightened sense of reality, (3) breach in the barriers of individuality, (4) inhibition of sense of repulsion, (5) release of sexual and moral tension, (6) delusions of grandeur and power, (7) sense of ineffable revelation.

A 'release of moral tension' sounds fantastic. Yes, please.

—

At the insistence of Reverend Canon LW Grensted, the former Nolloth Professor of the Philosophy of the Christian religion as a theologian with a deep interest in psychology, who had provided the foreword for the book, Custance wrote an afterword in which he describes Grensted tasking him with indicating his feelings, in a 'non-manic' state, towards the parts of the book written when manic. 'This is not very easy. The whole book is really the production of what I have called the "manic (or manic depressive) consciousness"' he writes before noting that 'some of the book was written in a state of at least relative "normality".' Custance is as confused as the rest of us about what 'normal' means to the manic depressive:

> Yet I am certainly not 'certifiable' now, whatever I may have been when I was actually certified in that instance. Why not? I am really just as 'mad' as ever. The difference is apparent rather than real. I just

do not appear to be 'mad', that is all. Certainly the apprehensions of the manic consciousness are as it were further away from my 'field of vision'.

In all truth, I pitched this book – successfully – while not 'normal' and was in a fairly dangerous, mixed-manic state. The start of the year had been tough for me, with a number of personal and professional conflicts that needed sorting through, and my brain simply couldn't process it and continue to operate at the same time. The upswing of all this was a hypomanic episode that came with its usual level of productivity. I wrote to the publisher of this book, reaching out to see if she would be interested in looking at a proposal from me. Reading back over the emails, I find them surprisingly lucid – this was a period largely of hypomania, not full-blown mania – but the tell tale signs are there: lack of anxiety, self-belief, a pinch of delusions of grandeur – and so it is clear that I have profited from my mania in this instance.

———

Repulsion and fascination seem to generate much of the wider public interest in mania. The actor Charlie Sheen raced through a 'fuck it all' breakdown in early 2011, after he was fired from his popular sitcom, the noxious *Two and a Half Men*, following a number of failed rehabilitation attempts. Sheen captivated audiences and entertainment journalists with outrageous grab quotes, saying he was a 'warlock' with 'tiger blood'. In an interview with American morning television journalist Andrea Canning, Sheen offered a cut-through expression – 'bi-winning' rather than bipolar – that caught on with the wider pop culture. Sheen's discomfort with the diagnosis would shift over time. Five years later, for an episode of the smarmy Oprah spin-off, *Dr Oz*, he sat in front of a live studio audience and submitted to an on-air psychiatric appointment to confirm his bipolar diagnosis. The psychiatrist was sheepish at first. She must have realised how unnatural this is to watch. Such a public therapy session might be of use, but I doubt it.

—

Why write this shit down at all?

—

'I told you I was ill' was Spike Milligan's desired epitaph, repeated throughout his life. He really did tell us he was ill.

—

In the opening pages of her memoir *Wishful Drinking*, Carrie Fisher includes a mock-up of the front page of the *Los Angeles Times* with the bold headline 'CARRIE FISHER SAYS: "I'M BIPOLAR"'. Celebrity culture is partly built on the demand for confession. The supermarket magazines are sold, adjacent to actual food, on such powerful hungers. The celebrity confessional – often co-authored, in some instances with a medical professional – takes hold soon enough. Spike Milligan was one of the first to go public with his diagnosis of manic depression. He was the one to wear it most outwardly – it was part of his public persona and drove the vocal innovations of *The Goon Show*. The public thrilled to such performances (later to be adopted by the likes of Robin Williams and Jim Carrey, both of whom have been associated with bipolarity). I watched clips of Milligan on YouTube – in the early days of its existence, aware of all the panic literature around its invention, pointing towards a fear of the narcissism it might engender in the young. One such video, uploaded in 2012, featured the Irish late-night talk show host Gay Byrne, explaining his decision to have Milligan on his show as a guest: 'As anyone who ever had anything to do with Spike could tell you, his mood could change very, very rapidly. So that when you invited Spike to the show, you didn't quite know which Spike you were going to get, because he could swing from being extrovert and funny and delightful and full of the joys of life to being somebody in a very, very bad mood.'

These confessionals, one by one, serve to add to a collective voice that actively works against stigma and discrimination. In riding rough waters, one needs a guide, or, at the very least, a guidebook.

There have always been books like these in my life, even if they disappeared, or were lost, or lent and never returned. A personal library can be eaten away, book by book, in a manic gifting spree. This was the case for others too. In her co-authored memoir-cum-self-help-guide *A Brilliant Madness: Living with Manic-Depressive Illness*, the actor Patty Duke describes being hospitalised following a period of severe mood swings, at the Cedars-Sinai Hospital in Los Angeles. There she was attended to by her psychiatrist and, wrote Duke, he placed a copy of the stage director Joshua Logan's book *Movie Stars, Real People and Me* in one of her hands, and her first lithium pill in the other. Logan, according to his *New*

York Times obituary, decided to come out about his manic-depression after being prescribed lithium at the end of the 1960s. Following that he 'took part in medical seminars, appeared on television and talked and wrote about his illness'. For Duke, then, confession and cure were grasped side by side, and perhaps the message from the doctor was that the confession itself was part cure.

—

In Leonard Michaels' *Sylvia*, a semi-autobiographical novella, partly constructed from cut-up journal entries, the author details his early marriage to the character of the title, and her death by suicide. I read it enthusiastically once, on my own. And the second time, I read it with my then girlfriend – my first long-term relationship – as we rode the train from Sydney to Newcastle. We sat next to each other and read the pages together – the only experience of tandem reading I've ever had. What did we want to know from this book? We wanted some explanation of what we were going through – a portrait of a couple, one of whom was sane and dealing with the other, who was most definitely out of their mind.

—

Mania as metaphor is used typically to imply free market impulses, out-of-control spending and over-consumption. This is mania as frenzied compulsion. Peter C Whybrow, after writing a practical text on mood disorders, went on to write *American Mania*, which built on his previous useful work as a basis for crafting metaphors damning the American psyche as a whole, and diagnosing the ills of its society. The book became a bestseller. In her near-ubiquitous essay

Illness as a Metaphor, written while undergoing treatment for cancer, Susan Sontag writes, as soberly as ever, that 'My point is that illness is *not* a metaphor, and that the most truthful way of regarding illness – and the healthiest way of being ill – is one most purified of, most resistant to, metaphoric thinking.' If 'illnesses have always been used as metaphors to enliven charges that a society was corrupt or unjust', as Sontag suggested, what do we make of Whybrow's use of mania as metaphor?

—

I was diagnosed at the age of twenty-two – and felt my first, and possibly strongest, mania then, in that year – as I finished a bachelor degree studying writing, and looked out at a life I didn't quite know how to handle. After being hospitalised, following a string of break-ins and other misdemeanours, I was sent to the Lawson Clinic in the suburb of Gordon, north of Sydney, which had just been opened. The clinic was named after the poet Henry Lawson. The poet was an appropriate namesake – he had suffered depression during his lifetime, and both he, his brother Peter and his mother, the criminally unrecognised suffragist and independent publisher Louisa Lawson, had been admitted to the nearby Callan Park Hospital for the Insane. The clinic itself was in a sterile single-storey house and nothing about it was intimidating. The psychiatrist was friendly and the only testing was a questionnaire on a computer.

As I waited for my appointment one morning, drinking bad coffee from McDonald's, I flipped through a tabloid newspaper – as junk as the food – when I came across a story that stood out. A woman was facing court for the murder of her husband, having stabbed him multiple times with an antique knife. The details were moreish but I couldn't read on because I had to get to the appointment. Later, reading the local broadsheet, I saw the same article; this time, however, I recognised the woman in the photograph. She was a classmate from university who I hadn't seen for a few years but who I used to sit next to and participated in group assignments with. The photograph in the tabloid had been taken from the time of her arrest – her face gazing downward, eyes tired from tears – whereas the broadsheet had run with a photograph outside the courthouse. They could have been two completely different people, and I only recognised one.

In the article, she was said to be suffering from borderline personality disorder – a term I had not registered before. She was eventually sentenced to four years' prison for manslaughter. I would see her at a writers' festival soon after, and it would take me an hour to realise who she was. I didn't know what to do with the information once it came to me.

—

In one of Joan Didion's most famous essays she uses a psychiatric report to attempt to convey the temperature of the times – the sticky paranoia of the end of the 1960s in California and elsewhere. The trick revelation in the title essay of *The White Album* is that the psychiatric report is her own, the result of a series of tests conducted at a private outpatient clinic in Santa Monica. She concludes her confession by noting wryly, 'By way of comment I offer only that an attack of vertigo and nausea does not now seem to me an inappropriate response to the summer of 1968.'

On reflection it is an infuriating use of mental illness as metaphor for the times. Didion was not suffering, she was just in tune, baby. But her influence is undeniable. The performativity of her disclosure would set the course for the personal essay for years to come. 'The patient to whom this psychiatric report refers to is me' could be the title for any number of memoirs.

—

I will not play that trick; instead I will be upfront with you. My latest report from my most recent GP, in the form of a referral to a psychologist and a mental health care plan, was something much shorter:

Personal history (eg childhood, education, relationship history, coping with previous stressors):

Close friend committed suicide 12 months ago
Another friend died of cancer 4 months ago
Recent high-level stress/conflict with colleagues he was living with
Episodes of racing thoughts, anger
Self-harm

Main problems/diagnosis (Risk/protective factors:
Bipolar disorder/recent self harm in context of severe stress)

Goal: Plan for curbing rage

—

American poetry in the middle of the twentieth century appeared to be a complex web of manic depressives, tied together like a cabal of spies, adding to each other's paranoia and offering various temptations. The literary critic Jeffrey Meyers wrote a group biography of these poets in *Manic Power: Robert Lowell and his Circle*; it is odd that Lowell takes the lead in the subtitle when the other poets (John Berryman, Theodore Roethke and Randall Jarrell) deserve equal billing. His epilogue concerns itself with Sylvia Plath – barely mentioned in the blurb for the book, as if she is an afterthought. Meyers is aware that the lives of poets that end in successful suicide take a certain place in the public imagination.

The disease could, as I have implied, be owned by literature. The trick is not mistaking it for an entry requirement for writing literature. The compulsive side of the condition – twinned with a collective competitiveness – led to so many confessional poetry breakthroughs. They wrote letters and dedicated poems to each other. They all seemed aware of each other's conditions. Lowell on Berryman: 'Hyper-enthusiasms made him a hot friend.' Delmore Schwartz: 'No one had John [Berryman]'s loyalty, but you like him to live in another city.'

Berryman had said in an interview: 'You ask me why my generation seems so screwed up? It seems they have every right to be disturbed. The current American society would drive anybody out of his skull, anybody who is responsive; it is almost unbearable. It doesn't treat poets very well.'

Robert Lowell, too, got it right when he said that it was 'some germ in the mind' but also 'There seems something generic about it.' It would be hard to avoid thinking this when in such proximity to so many friends going through the same thing. The lesson could be not to hang out with writers, but you can't always choose your friends, especially if you have to work in literary circles.

—

The editor Robert Giroux, of Farrar, Straus, Giroux, appeared in a public television documentary on Robert Lowell, as part of the aptly titled series *Voices & Visions*, musing on his author: 'The manic phases were not productive; whenever he went into a manic phase, he could not write. One of the most memorable statements in all the years I knew him was his saying that "It's terrible to think that all the suffering I have gone through and all the suffering I have caused was due to the fact that I didn't have enough salt in my brain."'

Salt in my brain.

That phrase stays with me.

—

In a short review of Redfield Jamison's long book on Robert Lowell, the cultural critic Julie Phillips questioned why that generation of American poets locked onto the imaginations of their fellow generation, asking: 'Why, at that moment, was there such an eager audience for their lunacy? Did the conservative citizens of the postwar years long for a channel to the mind of the mad? Did they want poets to be wild so they didn't have to? Or did they find personal pain less threatening than the voices of collective pain and anger that were struggling to make themselves heard?'

This goes to the heart of the boom in books about mental ill health. Looking over the titles on offer at the time, I can't help but question, was the culture-at-large bemused by all this or, in fact, somewhat obsessed? I got the feeling that part of it was giving in to the idea that life was too much, that we weren't really built for the contemporary moment. The popularity on writing about depression was really a validation of people's fragility. It was a breath out to read such things.

—

Nearly ten years after leaving the book behind in my adrenalin-fuelled run after being caught breaking into the beach house, and nearly ten years following my diagnosis as a manic-depressive, I finally tracked down another copy of *Broken Open*. Not the lost copy, but one stored in the University of Sydney library. I took it to a small wooden desk to inspect its contents. *Broken Open* was published in 2004 by the sports broadcaster Craig Hamilton, working with the ghostwriter Neil Jameson. My own psychotic episode took place just over an hour's travel away from the Newcastle train station where Hamilton had his. The book is ostensibly about his breakdown on his way to covering the 2000 Sydney Olympics for the national broadcaster. It is not very good, written in a blokey patter, with Jameson apparently trying to capture Hamilton's folksy Australian sing-song sports broadcaster voice, but the book is a decent basic introduction to the tenets of mania. Such books have their uses, but there is little literary pleasure to be found within them. Mania seems to elicit a rush towards mixed metaphors. In the space of a single paragraph Hamilton – or Jameson – compares mania to 'a major piece of space junk', a 'chain of detonations' and, then, a tsunami-size wave 'set to wipe out in awesome and truly awful style'. Michael Greenberg, in his memoir *Hurry Down Sunshine*, described the feeling of watching his daughter's manic episodes as 'being in the presence of a rare force of nature, such as a great blizzard or flood: destructive, but in its way astounding too'.

Bad weather abounds.

Why is it so easy to butcher the thinking about such a disorder? Is it because it invites extremes and so feels as if it requires extreme comparisons? Why not just describe it as a car, speeding until it stalls? In *Another Kind of Madness: A Journey Through the Stigma and Hope of Mental Illness*, the writer Stephen Hinshaw noted of his father's mania that: 'The engine continues to rev at a super-charged speed ...'

—

Broken Open does include chapters written from other perspectives, including those of Hamilton's wife, his best friend, a colleague and his psychiatrist. This might just be a way to fill out the pages, but it seems to be something of a trend. The collective commentary can also be found in the autobiography of the footballer Andrew 'Joey' Johns, whose wife wrote a chapter, and it included a contribution from the Knights' team physician. Johns counsels: 'I don't want to go on about it.' He says that the speaker tour circuit isn't for him, so why discuss the diagnosis at all? The discussion seemed to be part mea culpa for Johns, who had been caught in London's underground railway with ecstasy tablets on his person. He was issued with a caution, but was subsequently fed to the Australian tabloid media, who wanted immediate answers. So fucking what? People take ecstasy all the time. But Johns was the golden boy, and his fall needed a padded landing. So testimonials were needed to back up the confession. It's an incredibly sad read, and not just because it's so badly written.

—

At some point, it had occurred to me to do a much longer, Janet Malcolm–esque critical overview of memoirs about manic depression – in the style of her blistering rage against Sylvia Plath biographies in *The Silent Woman*, which in its strange way becomes the best biography of Sylvia Plath – but to sit above them seems disingenuous, and it is a problem I occasionally have with Malcolm as a writer. And I won't deny anyone their lived experience. I also just thought that I wasn't really interested in memoirs about manic depression or manic states, even though I am in the middle of writing one. I would like to think that this book goes against the grain.

—

I might have passed the point where books like these can be of any use to me. Should memoirs carry an expiry date? Still, the books certainly have their uses. Marya Hornbacher's *Madness: A Bipolar Life* contains a number of 'bipolar facts' and a list of website URLs in the back of her memoir. It shares part of its name with the Australian writer Kate Richards' *Madness: A Memoir*, along with a kind of diary-like structure. So, what, finally, after years of memoirs and medical accounts, is manic depression as a cultural identity?

—

Do I want this illness as such a stated and clear part of my identity? At the start of working on this book, when I would tell people what I was working on, I would shirk at mentioning the subject. 'It's not a memoir, more of a cultural look at mania – the manic side of manic-depression.' Why is it not a memoir? Because I'm embarrassed, I would reply. 'Those books are interesting, though,' an editor friend told me as we drove to a winter swim. Shouldn't that be the claim to stake – that the manic depressive is, by nature, a little *more* than you are, that I am a little more. But, as they say, more is less – and the more that comes along with mania will leave you with much, much less. I have to come to terms with the fact that the diagnosis is nefarious. It has not located something precise. It is not something that can be removed. It is an integral part of me. I just swing for the fences a little harder than most people.

—

Writing about illness has a powerful and useful cultural function. In *Intoxicated by My Illness*, Anatole Broyard writes, following his diagnosis with metastatic prostate cancer: 'The patient has to start by treating his illness not as a disaster, an occasion for depression or panic, but as a narrative, a story. Stories are antibodies against illness and pain.' And yet, I've also long carried with me the Roberto Bolaño quote, written while he was facing certain death from liver disease, 'Illness + Literature = Illness.'

4

RAPID THOUGHT GENERATOR: SAUL BELLOW'S *HUMBOLDT'S GIFT* AND KANYE WEST'S *THE LIFE OF PABLO*

1 What's weird in retrospect is how I seem to have willed some of these circumstances into being, how much I seemed to know before I knew anything at all. This came through reading too. As my first manic episode ratcheted up its peculiar intensity, giving me new, speedy ways of thinking, I bought a book by Saul Bellow from a secondhand store. Bellow had already become something of a talisman in my early writing life.

I had read *The Adventures of Augie March* while backpacking through Thailand the summer before – an uneasy match between book and location, but reader and time were simpatico. Bellow's energy and wide-eyed view of the world, making literature electric, awakened a great passion in me. I came home enthralled. Bellow had died a few years before in America, and was still receiving sombre notices and remembrances, but I, on the other hand, was just getting to the start of my life. I read *Seize the Day* on the train to Sydney, *Mr Sammler's Planet* on a couch near Newcastle, *The Dangling Man* looking over a beach in Wollongong, and *Herzog* in a Tasmanian youth hostel, in time for the first MOFO.

I took him with me wherever I went in my early twenties. *Humboldt's Gift* was something different from and more significant for me than these other novels though – a big, intimidating book, which I had heard much about through my critical readings.

To create the book Bellow had used the life of, and his friendship with, the American poet Delmore Schwartz as a subject for what is, in part, a hectic treatise on manic depression and the state of American life and poetry. The novel, published in 1975, goes some way to capturing the rapid, pulsing energy of someone experiencing mania, with a particular focus on the person's ability to leap between cultural references and connect thoughts, a way of thinking for which others may not have the capacity. The semi-autobiographical work opens, for instance, with Bellow's alter-ego, Charlie Citrine, taking a boat ride with the eponymous Delmore Schwartz substitute Von Humboldt Fleisher:

> On the ferryboat Humboldt said, 'I made it too young, I'm in trouble.' He was off then. His spiel took in Freud, Heine, Wagner, Goethe in Italy, Lenin's dead brother, Wild Bill Hickok's costumes, the New York Giants, Ring Lardner on grand opera, Swinburne on flagellation, and John D Rockefeller on religion.

All without taking much in the way of a breath, you imagine. This isn't just a case of being learned and knowing your history – having read the books, as such – it is rather a good example of the particular speed at which the mind goes when in manic mode. It is something like being stuck in top gear, unable to take your foot off the accelerator. It only gets real bad when the brake lines are cut, and usually you are the one who has cut them: self-sabotage can be added to the list of informal symptoms of this disorder.

Humboldt's Gift opens with Humboldt/Schwartz very much alive, talking at this speed, but Bellow really had no choice but to reveal the death of his subject early on in the piece – in the second chapter break – and to work backwards from there, piecing together his subject in relation to his premature demise.

2 I now own three copies of that novel – an original Viking hardback and a Penguin classic, which belong to my wife (a good sign for our relationship, that we share many similar interests), and a ratty paperback version I bought solely for the cover illustration – and, when drafting this paragraph, I could not locate a single one of them, because my house had become disordered, mirroring the state of my mind during the act of composition. The Viking hardback should have been visible to me, impossible to miss with its bright, gaudy yellow dust jacket. It had become an ominous object during my first episode of mania. I would see it lying around the house, and it would send me into a strange panic. I would start reading it, before jolting from my reading spot, and running around in circles five or six times. I didn't go quite so far as to consider this a demonic possession. It was just a book, but in that way it was scarier. It contained a lifetime of learning, everything that I hadn't read touched on in such a skipping manner. I didn't realise this was a symptom of the mania of Schwartz that Bellow was trying to get down. The book simply slayed me. (Bellow had this effect elsewhere and on others; Dave

Eggers has said that reading *Herzog* 'killed me when I was in my 20s' – 'killed me' is Bellovian language.)

The fact that I believed the book would send me mad was not incorrect, but was also, surely, part of the madness. Either way, I have never been able to locate again a quote that I believed came from Martin Amis about the book: that *Humboldt's Gift* was dangerous book to read in your twenties. As in, it would likely send you mad, or set you up for some intellectual failure, a portentous pratfall. The fact that I could not find the quote seemed to, in fact, prove its existence; that the book had, indeed, sent me around the bend because I had invented this quote that I would now forever be attempting to find in a looping literary quest. I like to think that Schwartz and his obsessive circular thinking would be proud somehow.

Did it start with a book? Would I have gone mad without a body of literature about madness sitting somewhere behind me, splayed open, many influential details contained within?

The obsession with a book was a sign of the disorder.

3 Bellow describes Humboldt/Schwartz thus: 'Poet, thinker, problem drinker, pill-taker, man of genius, manic depressive, intricate schemer, success story, he once wrote poems of great wit and beauty, but what had he done lately?' If I could quote the entire book, I probably would, and just provide annotations as my text.

4 Delmore Schwartz rose to prominence in the 1940s, following the publication of his first book *In Dreams Begin*

Responsibilities in 1938 at the age of twenty-four. The title story in that collection received rare praise from Vladimir Nabokov (who would later call Bellow a 'wicked wizard' and a 'miserable mediocrity') and appeared in the first issue of *Partisan Review*, which went on to become a defining 'little magazine' for the New York left-wing intelligentsia. Philip Rahv, one of the co-founders of that magazine, was, according to Schwartz, a 'manic-impressive'.

In this setting, Schwartz was introduced to aspiring poet John Berryman by the critic Mark Van Doren. Berryman and Schwartz became close, and discussed their ambitions for their careers. They were both hungry for success. Together, they schemed their way into teaching gigs. Schwartz served as a teacher and mentor to a young Lou Reed, who would later eulogise his former teacher in the first track of his comeback album *The Blue Mask* from 1982. Some have speculated that Reed too suffered bipolar, and his experience with ECT has been documented elsewhere.

Delmore Schwartz's unofficial nickname was The Heavy Bear, after his poem, 'The Heavy Bear Who Goes With Me' ('That heavy bear who sleeps with me/Howls in his sleep for a world of sugar'). And if Schwartz's life was one of an early rise to fame, it became one of early decline too, worthy of a retroactive inclusion in Samuel Johnson's *The Lives of the Poets*. The Heavy Bear rose to prominence alongside a new generation of American poets, many of whom would also suffer from manic depression. This group would worship at the altar of Eliot and Pound, and, by proximity to Pound, at that of madness too. Schwartz was the most vocal of the group in his support of Pound, having written a long essay to his 'useful labors' in a 1938 issue of *Poetry* magazine. Berryman visited the poet in the American psychiatric hospital he was transferred to in 1945 after his arrest for treason in Italy.

Pound was, of course, a foul anti-Semite, who did not deserve their love.

Schwartz's literary reputation has faded the way those of many poets do, but particularly in comparison with his contemporaries Lowell and Berryman, who have taken on mythic, Plath-like proportions, though that is largely down to the fact that they remained productive for a longer period. There have been many critical reassessments of Schwartz, including one by the great John Ashbery, published in the *New Yorker* in the year before Ashbery's death. Ashbery expressed a deep concern about Schwartz's contemporary reputation, and that James Atlas's biography *Delmore Schwartz: The Life of an American Poet* had overtaken the conversation (life cancelling out the poetry):

> The biography was a success not so much because people were at the time interested in Schwartz's poetry but because of the cautionary nature of his life story. Readers indifferent to modern poetry could still take grim relish in the classic saga of a brilliant poet, first heralded as a genius, the greatest young poet of his day, who quickly burnt himself out as a result of mental illness and addictions to alcohol and narcotics, and died almost forgotten at the age of fifty-two in a seedy hotel room in New York's Times Square district.

5 *Delmore Schwartz: The Life of an American Poet* intrigued readers at the time, but has largely been out of print in this

new century. It has undoubtedly been eclipsed by *Humboldt's Gift* as the go-to portrait of Schwartz's life. Bellow could have just as easily served as biographer. He was always there. He was the junior to this group but very much present. Like Schwartz, he had his first short story published in the *Partisan Review* at a young age. He was close to most of the figures within the group, and would later write the foreword to John Berryman's posthumously published semi-autobiographical novel *Recovery* – about Berryman's hospitalisations and periods in group analysis – and the two had been close friends. It was all grist for the mill. Bellow's latest biographer, Zachary Leader, believed that Berryman was also yoked in with the Humboldt portrait, used as a secondary source for Humboldt, although it is unclear what parts he would have contributed to a figure who is so wholly identified with Schwartz.

Bellow had long attempted to write about psychiatry, having completed a number of unpublished manuscripts about a fictionalised therapist. In Bellow's most recent biography, Zachary Leader's *The Life of Saul Bellow: To Fame and Fortune*, Leader tracked down an unpublished piece by Bellow in which he wrote that his own therapist 'and his room have been going round and round in my head for decades now. I can't say that I came away empty handed.'

As for Schwartz, he had taken Whitman's dictum from the epic 'Song of Myself': 'He most honors my style who learns under it to destroy the teacher', rendering the destruction literal. It appeared that he genuinely did believe that Bellow – amongst many others – was out to get him and do him in. The paranoid fantasies had truly taken over by the end of his life.

6 Saul Bellow was his own brand of weirdo though. In the novel he details Charlie Citrine's – and so his own – flirtation with Rudolf Steiner's theories of anthroposophy, with all its attendant spirits, echoing his own efforts to grapple with mysticism. It comes off just as mad as anything Humboldt experiments with. To pathologise Bellow is simply to return the serve. Perhaps Bellow had been touched by this kind of fire himself. This was the Bellow, after all, who had opened his 1964 novel *Herzog* with the infinitely quotable line: 'If I'm out of my mind, it's alright with me.' The quip was spoken by the title character Herzog; like Charlie Citrine, another in a long line of Bellow stand-ins in a career of quasi-autobiography.

So, what does it say that Citrine's big subject is 'boredom'? I don't think I have truly experienced boredom for years, certainly not since diagnosis, say. There was the influence of parental discipline: 'If you're bored, pick up a tea towel.' But can the manic depressive mind encounter boredom? Depression or melancholia are not the same as boredom – the mind is active or inactive, but attention is not taken away completely.

7 Reading is a dangerous act and a hazardous art. Empathy, which reading engenders, is a fickle creature. Bellow wrote in the short story 'Him With His Foot in His Mouth', 'Human beings can lose their lives in libraries. They ought to be warned.' If you can lose your life in a library, you can gain one too. Reading can be good, of course, for building character. From the start of wanting to write and wanting to be a writer (sometimes different ambitions, sometimes the same), there were books that did this for me. And there were the

lives of writers, as mapped out by biographers, and sometimes themselves.

Reading has also provided a way to form kinship. The memoirs sit beside me now in a pile, and no matter their quality, at least they say: 'Yes, this condition exists. My experiences are broadly yours'.

I was not yet manic when I enrolled in a writing degree at the age of eighteen, or so, but I soon would be. The twentieth century is littered with literary figures who stumbled into some form of madness. It has become a marker of a kind of literary marketplace. And for a young writing student, it provided a bipolar bibliography. So while others dangerously romanticised melancholia, I was smitten with mania. I was reaching out for writers like Richard Yates, whose suffering seemed to colour their writing, and their world. Before reading about Humboldt, for instance, I had, in my first year at university, discovered and devoured *The Collected Stories of Richard Yates* – quite a few years before the Richard Yates renaissance had swung into our lives due to a film adaptation of one his novels, *Revolutionary Road*, being released. It is less his stories that stay with me now, than Blake Bailey's big bold biography *A Tragic Honesty: The Life and Work of Richard Yates*. In here, were the first descriptions of bipolarity that I had likely come across, and they soothed me. It's bad aspirational literature to have around at an impressionable age. It is an ongoing problem for literature as 'industry'. When writing is seen as a calling, rather than a profession, problems can arise. The biography of a writer is extra-literary – it extends the creative work, or attempts to explain it away.

It was the first case, for me, of identifying with the life as much as the writing. Ordering the book from an American website, I did not know what was coming, or why I wanted to read about his life. I probably wanted to know, most of all, how he had done it. The stories were good. This was something to aspire to. Instead, I got a map to a life of destitution and constant rejection (Yates was tortured by the fact that he never had a short story accepted by the *New Yorker* in his lifetime). I was captivated by Bailey's description of one of Yates's many breakdowns:

> Yates was drinking too much, perhaps in an effort to mitigate the rampant pangs of mania – the exhilaration and paranoia, the sense of being stared at and discussed. Yates finally erupted into full-blown, roaring-drunk psychosis at Treman Cottage, where he seems insistently to have helped himself to other people's liquor … Ultimately he thought he was becoming the Messiah (a common delusion of mania), and legend has it he clambered onto the roof of Treman and held out his arms as though crucified. He told Grace Schulman he remembered swinging from tree branches and naming his gawking students after Christ's disciples, though it's hard to imagine someone with Yates's stamina exerting himself to that extent.

This was a bad influence for a young student of writing, a terrible model to stare at. I sat in class patiently waiting for my outburst. When would I go mad, how could I misbehave on the same level? When it did come, it hit hard.

The resurgence and revival of Richard Yates's work prompted by Sam Mendes' film adaptation of *Revolutionary Road* provided an opportunity for a public reckoning with mania, but it didn't quite happen. The film was received as a historical document, rather than something that represented the urgent mental health struggles of multiple characters. Suddenly paperbacks with the concerned – constipated – acting-faces of Leonardo DiCaprio and Kate Winslet on the front cover were widely available. Michael Shannon earned an Oscar nomination for his wacky performance. One wonders if any lessons were really learnt.

8 There is a small, yet significant, moment in *Humboldt's Gift*, which has grown ever more present in my mind, and which has come, for me, to define everything about how others look at mania. Two months before Humboldt's death, Charlie spies him in the street. From behind a parked car, Charlie watches the poet eat a pretzel stick, something of a destitute street lunch, and decides not to approach his old friend, largely because 'he had death all over him'. Charlie, that day, had been living the high life – travelling around New York in a helicopter with the coast guard and Senator Robert Kennedy for a magazine profile (this was taken from life, literally; Bellow was commissioned by *Life* magazine to cover the potential presidential candidate in 1966). The ignominy of the snub is partly that it is never directly received. This occurs twice over. Firstly, in the book, Humboldt never sees Charlie and cannot rectify the situation, not being aware that it has even occurred (such is often the case with such social damnations). Then Bellow wrote it up in his novel – in which Humboldt is so very obviously Schwartz – and Schwartz wasn't alive to read it. Delmore Schwartz died in 1966, aged just fifty-two; Bellow published

Humboldt's Gift nine years later in 1975. Bellow, having out-lived Schwartz and then some, had the advantage of hind-sight that Schwartz would never be afforded.

Later in the book, Bellow self-corrects, writing, 'I had run away from him on Forty-sixth Street just when he had the most to tell me.' He does not quite regret his decision to avoid Humboldt, but he notes, seriously, the transgression on his behalf. To turn away is a great injustice.

9 Mania – via its many behavioural extremes – creates a severe isolating effect; where depression might mean that you push people away on your own terms, mania screams at people to fuck off – get the fuck out, get the fuck away from me – as an involuntary consequence of its symp-toms. Who wants to be around real-life lunacy? Who wants to put themselves at risk of theft, harassment, potential vio-lence, mean-spiritedness and plain idiocy? No one is saying it is an easy thing to be around. *Humboldt's Gift* is a good tes-tament to this. It paints a picture of Schwartz's growing par-anoia, and his sharp lashings – largely in letters, sometimes in person. He sent brutal missives and threatened those clos-est to him with court filings. There were bitter fallings-out, which were conflict driven and typically one-sided. This is the fate of the manic depressive, overly prone to such para-noiac flame-outs.

10 I experienced this side of mania as I turned thirty. In 2015, in the middle of my second manic episode, I began a concerted effort to uncover the make-up of the Book

Council of Australia. I sat out in an open-air bar in Huskisson, writing a letter to the Prime Minister, asking for information on how the group had been formulated and its purposes. I called for the resignation of its inaugural chair, and then, in a moment of inspiration, sought the co-signature of Nick Cave ('He's a writer too!'). Cave sent a statement through an intermediary: 'Many truly gifted Australian writers are struggling, writers of vision and vitality. This need not be the case. Writers, like other artists, are the lifeblood of a nation, those bold few who dare reflect us back to ourselves, in all our beautiful ignobility.', So, newly thirty, I went after the Minister for the Arts with zeal, and a particular arsenal, writing a piece I published in the *Sydney Morning Herald* with the support of such high-profile signatories as Nick Cave and JM Coetzee, demanding to know why funding had been directed away from the Literature Board of the Australia Council. This campaign turned into a three-month endeavour, working around the clock without pay, which left me exhausted but also manic, overstimulated by the volume of correspondence. I was convinced I had enemies, and maybe I did.

11 There are further examples of degradation to be found, and often their traditional site is the psychiatric hospital: arrested and taken to the very real Bellevue Hospital, Humboldt suffers diarrhoea and is locked away 'in a state of filth'. (Did this happen to Schwartz? If not, what is the point of inventing the shit?) Bellow writes: 'I understood what emotions had torn at Humboldt's heart when they grabbed him and tied him up and raced him to Bellevue. The man of talent struggled with cops and orderlies. And, up against the

social order, he had to fight his Shakespearian longing, too – the longing for passionate speech.'

Psychiatric hospitals take up a peculiar space in the public imagination. They represent the end of a line for some – the ultimate sign of a breakdown in a person's control over their own lives. Their depiction in films and books have provided many with a morbid portrait of what happens inside their walls. *One Flew Over the Cuckoo's Nest* delivered an interesting view: a relatively sane person is admitted and is subjected to the worst of hospitalisation nightmares, forced lobotomies probably chief amongst them.

I would only ever be kept in a psychiatric ward for two nights. This followed my attempted break-in at the beach. My father called an ambulance, which took me to the local emergency department where I was looked over (I had one physical symptom, a swollen ankle resulting from kicking a wall). The doctors gave me the all-clear and sent me home. As soon as I got there, I started trying to get down to the beach to break into the house again, and so my father called the police, and it was straight back to the hospital – where the attending doctors finally admitted that, yes, I should be admitted. The ward I was escorted to felt cordoned off from the rest of the hospital – a security measure, which gave the place the feel of a sanctuary. I was behind safe enough walls for now. Maybe it would be good for me? Saul Bellow had suggested John Berryman had 'found his society' in such places. I shuddered at the thought of becoming too attached to such a place, but it had its comforts. This was where you were told to stop. The brakes were put on for you. It was a relief. Rest was necessary and prescribed, but not rest alone. Being drugged in a white room with nothing in it wasn't real rest. The antipsychotic I had been given on arrival meant I couldn't keep my eyes open for very long and soon I was going at the pace of a coma patient. They locked the book I had brought with me in a drawer. That seemed counter-productive, as reading had been the only thing that had managed to keep me still in the last months.

When I woke up, in a stupor I explored what was outside my room. The TV screen in the common area kept playing the same scene of a water skier over and over. He was trapped in perpetual motion. I realised that I had stopped watching television over the summer, except for the tennis, and that this maybe explained the state my mind was in. Maybe everyone needed television now to keep them on the level deemed sane. There were tea and coffee making facilities – they trusted you with hot water! – and cold store-bought sandwiches in plastic wrap. Salmon, tuna and salad. They were delivering us our omega 3 covertly. Later they would ask that I take ten fish oil tablets at once; I would burp up the bottom of the ocean all night. I had three salmon sandwiches and then went and looked outside at the courtyard. It was walled in by bricks that went twenty metres high. There was a girl who looked no more than fifteen, smoking on a bench. She brought her legs up and rested her chin on her knees. The security camera on the top of the wall seemed to watch her more closely than I did.

Back inside, beside the television, were pamphlets with titles such as 'Bipolar and You' – that made it sound like schizophrenia, as if the bipolar was a separate personality. I kept watching that water skier.

I was given a pink pill to put on my tongue and it was lights out.

The nurse stirred me awake the next morning. I had an appointment in the next room with the resident psychiatrist, who was in his late seventies. I could not keep my head up as he asked his questions. His conclusion, which came after only one day of observation, was that there was nothing mentally wrong with me; I was only angry with my parents for not letting me take the car out for the night.

It is worth noting that I wasn't in there for long. Partly this relates to the function a psychiatric hospital plays in a manic episode – there to make an attempt to cease and treat the behaviour that has led one there. Medical narratives aren't my territory. Many other books on manic depression contain at least one treatise on the ethics of treating the disease with pharmaceuticals, but this isn't one of them.

I wasn't quite psychotic, I guess. I remained lucid enough to convince the doctors that I should be sent home in the first place, and a gift of the gab helped keep me there. In manic episodes, more than anything I was a con artist convincing others of my relative sanity.

12 Of the manic depressive poets I've been drawn to, the writing of others who surrounded them provide more insightful commentary than the poets themselves. Eileen Simpson, whose first husband was John Berryman, painted a sensitive portrait of the scene in her memoir *Poets in Their Youth*. Simpson outlived most of her male contemporaries and went on to become a psychologist, writing other autobiographies-as-social-studies, one on overcoming dyslexia and one on marriage in later life. Simpson detailed lovingly the early friendship of Berryman and Schwartz, but the book

had to turn somewhat darker, as did their lives. By the end, the author was surveying a sombre scene: 'Ted was not in his right mind. Cal, in Salzburg, had gone clear out of his again'. Simpson is particularly distraught at Schwartz's disintegration. Like Bellow before her, she spies Schwartz out in the world, in this instance scrambling to catch a train. His appearance worries her – 'hair wild, clothes in disorder' – and she notes his pallor and nervous energy. Unlike Bellow, she acknowledges him and they sit on the train together. Simpson can't tell if he wants to talk or not, but comes to realise that Schwartz can no longer listen. She finally observes, 'Delmore had changed so heartbreakingly one could no longer use the word "crazy" in the old innocent way when talking about him.'

In the very next sentence, after going through her list of diagnosed manic depressives, she drops: 'Saul was sane.'

Somehow that Bellow is diagnosed as 'sane' hurts most of all. How do some come out of all of this alive?

13 Part of the illness will always involve a certain removal of autonomy; if part of the self is transfigured by it, part of your agency is lost. You have to give up certain things. At your lowest, this can mean practically everything. Witness is important too, but what happens when one person runs away with the story, and takes the credit for its creation? Schwartz was not alone in being turned into fiction by Bellow. There were the ex-wives, family members, romantic competitors, fellow novelists, critics and academics. The canvas, for Bellow, was wide because it was made up of multitudes. People felt used, chewed up. The academic David Mikics wrote an entire book dedicated to

the subject, titled *Bellow's People: How Saul Bellow Made Life into Art*. Mikics' book gets to the heart of Bellow's transgressions in transcribing someone's very being – their life – into the fictional arena. Indeed, Bellow made an entire career out of other people's lives. The great writer vacuumed up people and the details of their lives all throughout his writing career, until the very end (his final book, *Ravelstein*, about the academic Allan Bloom, another big talker, hews close to *Humboldt's Gift* and has Ravelstein, the Bloom stand-in, practically persuading Bellow to write his biography, which of course becomes the book in question).

It's not as if famous manic depressives did not do ransacking of their own (most famously Robert Lowell used his ex-wife Elizabeth Hardwick's personal letters to construct the poems in *The Dolphin*). Bellow, however, ultimately controls the narrative. Madness provides a great generative plot engine – the systems set for a rise and fall, a cache of narrative gold. Bellow, never having been really enamoured by the idea of plot, resisted such straightforward structure, instead turning Humboldt into something more of a reflective memoriam in motion.

14 Bellow isn't known for his dialogue. However, he reportedly dictated large parts of the novel into a recording device while pacing his office, before having it transcribed by someone else. So, in one sense, the novel is all monologue. It's long but Bellow has always been associated with excess; his breakthrough with *The Adventures of Augie March* was one of a flow of language, embracing everything and replicating the rapid patter of street talk for high art purposes.

Bellow seemed to understand, innately, the symptoms of mania and used them to drive his fictions. He had a powerful conception of the way the mind can skip, and speed ahead, with racing thought. In an iconic scene in *Seize the Day*, Bellow has his main character connect a glass of water through all of history. Looking at the table in front of him, he is gripped by the glass:

> If you wanted to talk about a glass of water, you had to start back with God creating the heavens and earth; the apple; Abraham; Moses and Jesus; Rome; the Middle Ages; gunpowder; the Revolution; back to Newton; up to Einstein; then war and Lenin and Hitler. After reviewing this and getting it all straight again you could proceed to talk about a glass of water.

Is Herzog, based on Bellow, in the grips of a seeming case of hypergraphia, any worse off mentally than Humboldt, based on Schwartz? By novel's end Herzog has crashed his car, and soon enough gives up the letter writing. Schwartz was rendered a tragic figure in life, but he is a largely comic figure in *Humboldt's Gift*. Does the manic depressive become life's ultimate tragi-comic persona?

15 What is Humboldt's gift? The eponymous gift is, in the end, an outline for a film. Bellow's gift to him in return is a proper plot, in the other sense of the word. A plot for a plot; he reburies Humboldt with his mother. The film treatment is, ultimately, unusable and mostly nonsense. This fits with the character's ultimate fate and the sense of destitution, that of lost promise.

16 *Humboldt's Gift* becomes an early quotation in Kay Redfield Jamison's *Touched with Fire* – Redfield Jamison quotes a grab of speech about 'Henry Adams, Henry James, Henry Ford …' – and perhaps people now come to the novel with the same set of references in mind. Certainly, I have mined them here. Redfield Jamison describes the book as 'one of the best descriptions of the far-ranging, intoxicating and leapfrogging nature of manic thought and conversation'. Why exactly this way of thinking translates into creativity – and the act of getting that elusive, jumpy thought into a concrete scribing – is something she explores at length. Writing is thought's translation, the act of making it real and ready to broadcast out of the head. There is a compulsive element – another driving feature of mania – that writers possess above all others. We can't help ourselves.

17 'Thought is made in the mouth. I still consider myself very likeable,' Tristan Tzara proffers in his *Dada Manifesto on Feeble Love and Bitter Love*. Talk is compulsive for the manic depressive. Bellow quotes the owner of a restaurant Schwartz was known to frequent: 'That guy will talk your head off'. Manic speech is called 'pressured speech' by psychologists. Emil Kraepelin, writes Kay Redfield Jamison, 'observed that manic speech was a type to itself and that its characteristic pacing and sounds tied it to rhyme and free associative speech'.

18 Bellow writes of Schwartz: 'He was a great entertainer but going insane. The pathologic element could be

missed only by those laughing too hard to look.' The same could be written of the rapper Kanye West today. Throughout 2016, West teased the release of his next album, which would eventually come to be titled *The Life of Pablo*. Through Twitter he provided both constant updates and bold brags about the quality of the work. The social media platform provided an unparalleled view into the psyche of an artist working on a large-scale ultra-hyped project. The final track on the eventuating album, 'Saint Pablo', narrates this in a meta-narrative that unfolds like a sustained autobiography of the making of the record. He sing-speaks that people on Twitter are trying to send him crazy. He wisely identifies ownership of one's own narrative as the key to mental wellbeing. In one of the best lines on the album he implies that the perception of him is wrong: he is not out of control, he is simply out of the control of others.

West had much to contend with which was out of his control. Early that year, *Rolling Stone* published an opinion piece with the headline: 'Kanye West may be crazy, but he's still important to rap culture'. There are more examples of this brand of dangerous armchair psychologist commentary.

Throughout his career West had risen to even greater heights of fame and with it, infamy, the two going hand in hand: an ascendant trajectory made literal by his live performances in late 2016, in which he performed on an elevated stage, constructed, one can only imagine, to capture his larger-than-life personality. He hovered directly above his audience, suspended in the air. West has certainly adopted some of John Lennon's bravado when it comes to Christ-like symbolism and shares a fondness for equating himself with Jesus. So, part of his character has always centred around delusions of grandeur. Of course, West is talented enough to substantiate such claims. But even truth and reality have their own delusional element – fame, at the level experienced by West, can only heighten these experiences.

It was on this elevated platform at one performance in Sacramento that West seemed to give in fully, and finally, to the delusions. Again, the new age of ubiquitous camera technology built into our phones allowed the moment to be captured and published within seconds of it occurring. After that performance – or *anti-performance* – in Sacramento West was hospitalised. He had good reason to be put under such care. His wife, the global celebrity Kim Kardashian, had been robbed at gunpoint in her supposedly secure Paris hotel room. External stressors are often underreported in instances of mania, but they were clear in West's 2016 timeline.

For years West broke social conventions – snatching the microphone from Taylor Swift to correct the record at the 2009 VMAs that, indeed, Beyonce should have won Best Female Video – and many of us applauded his transgressions, even if we squirmed or disagreed with his actions. We ate it up, as they say. Resistance was part of his brand identity. The pathological element underneath all of this wasn't left unexamined, but somehow it wasn't quite fully in view. Up on his platform, West showed us just how pathological things can really get. West's speech, and the speed at which his mind was free associating, entered a literary and rhetorical space that is usually only found in the essayistic dialogue of the novels of a DeLillo or a Pynchon. It carries the paranoid quality of those writers too. It certainly acts as a Bellow-like monologue, running rampant through cultural touchstones, and trying to express a big-picture view of the world.

Bellow writes in *Seize the Day* that 'You were lucky even … to make yourself understood. And this happened over and over and over with everyone you met. You had to translate and translate, explain and explain, back and forth, and it was the punishment of hell itself not to understand or be understood.' West, in his contemporary moment, surely lives, and struggles, with 'the punishment of hell itself not to understand or be understood'. Part of his critical thinking is defensive on this level. He wants to be understood but doesn't trust that people follow his logic. Rapid speech often fills the space where the person experiencing mania feels that others' understanding should be; overplaying and over-explaining their position in the world in opposition to others. Give a man an elevated platform, and he will likely use it in this way.

19 Has there ever been an artform that has come any-where near as close to capturing spontaneous speech – the oncoming bullet train of thought transcribed in real time – as rap, particularly in its freestyle mode? Rap isn't simply the freeform creation of spoken-word lyrics, however; it's also an extremely complex construction of beats, and frequently, sam-ples. The successful use of samples requires a skilful ability to free associate and jump between ideas and cultural history – to seek out an existing musical source, often obscure, that serves the song being written. In fact, a fantastic way to unearth music you haven't heard is to work in reverse from a rap song using a sample. West, who received his first sampler at the age of fifteen, began his career as a producer for other artists, working his way up to his breakthrough efforts on Jay-Z's *The Blueprint*. Part of West's enormous talent is the quickness of his mind in both his musical and literary vocabulary. Rap relies, in part, on humour and wordplay. Speed is prized, too. Bravado is important to

the constructed identity of the mainstream rapper. A sort of back and forth bragging and attacking is expected between contemporaries. Delusions of grandeur are common ground. All arguably signs pointing towards a form of forceful mania.

20 More concerning to me than watching Kanye West's meltdown at the short-lived Sacramento concert was his appearance on the ultra-innocuous daytime TV program *Ellen*, hosted by the beloved Ellen DeGeneres. Perhaps it pointed to what would later occur in Sacramento. West's interview spun out of control. What is hard to reconcile here is that he is indeed very talented: one of the world's greatest producers of rap music. But he's not a particularly interesting fashion designer, and here he was on *Ellen*, talking about the genius of his work in fashion. He jumps up and down in a manner reminiscent of Tom Cruise's infamous couch leaping on *Oprah*, eleven years prior. West's 'MASSIVE rant' (as YouTube uploaders phrased it) was impossible to interrupt, and Ellen sat in silence, bearing witness in nervous bemusement. His appearance on the program, which was aired on 19 May 2016, almost felt like a performance piece, although his remarks were certainly just off-the-cuff interview banter, though the triviality of the relaxed couch question and answer format was certainly taken to strange extremes. I transcribe one of his answers here, almost in full, despite how marred and ugly it will make the literary quality of this work appear:

> Picasso is dead. Steve Jobs is dead. Walt Disney is
> dead. Name somebody living that you can name in the

same breath as them. Don't tell me about being likable.
We got 100 years here. We're one race, the human
race, one civilization. We're a blip in the existence of
the universe, and we constantly try to pull each other
down. Not doing things to help each other. That's my
point. It's like I'm shaking talking about it. I know it's
daytime TV, but I feel I can make a difference while
I'm here. I feel that I can make things better through
my skill set. I am an artist. Five years old, art school
Ph.D, Art Institute of Chicago. I am an artist. I have a
condition called synesthesia where I see sounds. I see
them. Everything that I sonically make is a painting.
I see it. I see the importance in the value of everyone
being able to experience a more beautiful life. When
I make clothes … It's funny because I'll sit there with
Obama and Leo's talking about the environment and
I'm talking about clothes and everyone looks at me
like, 'That's not an important issue.' But I remember
going to school in fifth grade and wanting to have
a cool outfit. I called the head of Payless. I'm like,
'I want to work with you. I want to take all this
information that I've learned from sitting in all these
fashion shows and knocking on all these doors and
buying all these expensive clothes, and I want to take
away bullying.' Michael Jackson and Russell Simmons
is [sic] the reason I was able to go so far in music.
There was a time when Michael Jackson couldn't get
his video on MTV because he was considered to be
'urban'. The Michael Jackson. So I literally have to be
the Michael Jackson of apparel in order to break open
the doors of everyone that will come after I'm gone.

After I'm dead. After they call me 'Wacko Kanye'.
[crowd laughter] Isn't that so funny? That people
point fingers at the people who have influenced us the
most. They talk the most shit about the people who
cared the most. I'm sorry daytime television. I'm sorry
for the realness.

With West listing off Picasso, Jobs, Walt Disney, Michael
Jackson and (most strangely of all) Russell Simmons, how
can this not remind one of Von Humboldt Fleisher's style of
verbal mind-mapping? 'It's not daytime television any more,'
Ellen quips at the end of this monologue, pleasing the audience immensely. She's right, of course. The conversation has
diverted from the usual protocol. What is it if not daytime
television, then? Mania can test the patience of those around
it, but on a stage in front of a live audience, it provides much
entertainment value. West's thought explosions occurred
online too, and his constant tinkering with *Pablo* pointed
towards a level of perfectionism rarely displayed in such a
public way. Expectations were high, but people also thrilled
to the chaos of it all.

No one was expecting just how autobiographical it would
all become when it came to his psychological troubles. On
the track 'FML' (a popular abbreviation for Fuck My Life),
he raps about living without limits and going off the drug
Lexapro. West had previously mentioned the drug when he
featured on the track 'U Mad' by Vic Mensa, rapping that it
left him drowsy, and felt, to him, like a heart attack (one of
the side-effects of Lexapro is heartburn). Lexapro is typically
used to treat depression and anxiety, but can be used in treating bipolar disorder. Like many antidepressants, Lexapro

can activate underlying mania. The Weeknd provides the chorus for the track in which he laments, seeming to envy Kanye's self-destructive tendencies, that he wishes he could fuck his life up. The pull of self-destruction is all too familiar to the manic depressive. A heavily autotuned voice – to the point of feeling automated – tempts the singers to throw all their cares away. On the track 'No More Parties in LA' he talks of seeing a psychiatrist and taking Xans (short for the pharmaceutical Xanax).

There has to be some meaning in the fact that he put two tracks back to back titled 'Low Lights' and 'Highlights'. The titles speak to each other – the bipolar poles – if not their actual content.

On 'Feedback' he demands that the listener give him the name of one genius who isn't crazy.

21 Why have pop stars melting down become the most mythologised cases of mania? Brian Wilson, might be the prime example, and Michael Jackson dangling a baby named Blanket out of a window in Berlin comes to mind too, but there are a number of young female pop singers making up the majority: Demi Lovato, Lindsay Lohan, Amanda Bynes, Britney Spears. Lovato is the only one who has been public about a diagnosis of bipolar disorder. There is a strong case for suggesting that environmental stress factors are greater for these women. To have everyone talking about you, wanting a photo with you, to hug you, tell you they love you, is a recipe for overstimulation. The same goes, of course, for Jason Russell slapping the pavement nude, his arsehole blurred out by TMZ's editors: everyone was talking about his video, debating the ethics of it, or sending millions of

messages of support for the cause. Attention on a mass scale can be highly traumatic.

22 In 2017 the Australian music festival Splendour in the Grass ran into a controversy on announcing that the Spanish art collective Hungry Castle would be featuring a sculpture titled *Sad Kanye*. Essentially a giant floating head – a ten-metre inflatable – the sculpture was criticised for not taking seriously, and, indeed, making light of, Kanye West's struggles with mental ill health during his life, which had intensified in the space of that year. Hungry Castle released a statement shortly after, reading:

> It was never our intention to start a dialogue about mental health issues. But as you know more than anybody, great art can often be divisive and is ultimately open to the interpretation of the public. We want to thank the internet for opening our eyes to this viewpoint and we now see how this project could be viewed as insensitive.

The group relented and decided to rename the artwork *Happy Kanye*.

23 In *How Literature Saved My Life*, the American writer David Shields writes about the fall and sudden disgrace of Tiger Woods, following his car crash and the details to follow about marital indiscretions. Shields muses on his obsession about stories of such celebrity revelations:

When my difficult heroes (and all real heroes are difficult) self-destruct, I retreat and reassure myself that it's safer here close to shore, where I live ... I want the good in my heroes, the gift in them, not the nastiness, or so I pretend. Publicly, I tsk-tsk, chasting their transgressions. Secretly, I thrill to their violations, their (psychic or physical) violence, because through them I vicariously renew my shadow side.

Delmore Schwartz and Kanye West – or Humboldt and Yeezy – now form and inform so much of my thinking that they walk with me, as I work my way through this world. So, Delmore and Kanye, I commune with your lives, defer to you, and, through this, renew my shadow side. It's dark out here with you, but you invariably light the path.

24 On his release from psychiatric care, West dyed his hair blond. There seemed to me, on looking at the photographs of Kanye with his new hair, casually reclining, in a West Hollywood gallery, that there was a convergence, in the phrase often used by the nonfiction writer Lawrence Weschler. An echo. To wit: it reminded me immediately of Britney Spears' shaved head, during her troubles in 2007 and 2008. Why should these hair changes signify anything to do with mental ill health, other than the fact that they coincided with the timing of these superstar crises? In Spears' case, a woman with a shaved head appears to the culture at large to be a radical act – a defiance and a resistance in itself. This seems wrong for any number of gendered reasons, a judg-mental populace shaming the star for daring to simply change

her look (something they demand of stars all the time in fashion magazines and commentary).

25 On *Blond(e)*, Frank Ocean sings to an unidentified 'you' on the track 'Self Control' that they have lived a 'blonded life'. I could not help, looking at the post-hospitalisation photographs of West, wondering if he had listened to that record too many times, and was trying to enact it in real time. What is a 'blonded life'? A life lived too bright? I recall the Saul Bellow gag, 'She was a suicide blonde, dyed by her own hand.' The blaring white of peroxide is a political statement of a sort and to conform to the messages of a song called 'Self Control' is a political act. West knew what he was doing. I hope West knew what he was doing. I think West knew what he was doing. I'm pretty sure West knew what he was doing. I think I know what I'm doing. I hope I know what I'm doing. I'm not sure if I know that what I'm doing relates to West at all. I hope there is a shared way of thinking of the world with some, with West, with Ocean, with Spears, with Bellow, with Herzog, with Humboldt, with Reed, with Schwartz, with others. Take me to the river of similar feeling and same thought.

WAYS
OF
SEEING

5

IT'S JUST TOO FUCKING *TOO*: MANIA IN CINEMA AND THE FILMS OF PAUL THOMAS ANDERSON

It's a *lot*, sometimes. Like, a *lot*.

—

Cinema is excess – that's the short of it.

—

In the incredible making-of documentary for the film *Magnolia* – a video diary released as a DVD extra, but a one-hour and then some film in its own right – Paul Thomas Anderson is seen doing a strange dance with a woman who embodies his film. He berates her for being too long, and being unloved compared to earlier efforts, and he reflects pointedly, 'It's all just too fucking *too*'.

—

The long of it: cinema is the art of excess and I felt this keenly when coming out of a major depressive episode and reckoning with an oncoming mania. When I was depressed for the last time – and let's say that we hope we keep it at that – I thought I would never live to see New York, and then, suddenly,

I was in New York. I didn't think I would ever see New York because at the start of that year I was depressed, convinced I was going to die some time that year, so I was going through the list of things I would never do that I thought I should. But then, yeah, I was in New York, on travel funding from the UNESCO Melbourne City of Literature office and I still wasn't quite well – a paranoid edge remaining in action – but I was glad to see a city of such epic mythology, and I was thinking a lot about film, because I knew the city largely from cinema. I also really just wanted to go and see movies while in the city, because it seemed like such a movie-going city. If LA makes them, NY consumes them. Nothing I can say is right about the city, but maybe there are no wrong answers. So, I saw and loved *Love & Mercy* in the middle of New York in the middle of their summer, in a little cinema complex, somewhere within walking distance of the Guggenheim Museum, after having had a panic attack after leaving the gallery. I suppose if I were to diagnose it, I had the effects of agoraphobia: I could not look skyward, as I believed the sky, acting in a conspiracy with Manhattan's sleek skyscrapers, was going to suck me up and spit me out into the cold void of space (a fear largely born of the twisting cityscapes of Christopher Nolan's *Inception* and misguided repeated viewings of the footage of the World Trade Center towers falling to the earth on 11 September 2001; you can throw in a confused reading of Don DeLillo's fiction, particularly *Falling Man*, for good measure). So I spent a lot of time looking at my shoes that day, and my wife insisted we find refuge in a cinema, to escape the midsummer heat and the heat within my head. Why not watch a film about some of the mental health issues you yourself are struggling with? The movie hit me in the gut, and by its end, I was in tears. The film closes with the ageing, real-life Brian Wilson performing the title song *Love & Mercy*. For the rest of our time in New York, I was humming its melody to the point where the real danger wasn't some sudden space vortex, but my newlywed wife killing me out of pure frustration with having to hear the song over and over and over and over and over and over and over and over and over and over and over and over and over and over and over and over and over and over and over again.

—

Love & Mercy, directed by the film producer Bill Pohlad – the son of a billionaire owner of a baseball team (how's that for fucking nuts?) – documents the life of the key figure of beloved pop band The Beach Boys, Brian Wilson. The film charts both his early career creating the sonic masterpiece *Pet Sounds* and struggle to complete the lost record *Smile*. The film was produced with authorisation from Wilson, and, with an uber-honesty, documents his recovery from a post-*Smile* over-medicated fugue state. Pohlad splits the film in two – and cast different actors in the role of Brian Wilson – and this decision, critically, does not feel like just a storytelling device. Rather, it appears to be a strategic decision to access the core effects of manic depression, as lived by Wilson. The young actor Paul Dano plays Brian Wilson when he is up – in a creative purple patch, writing songs at a rapid rate, before his fall – whereas a washed-out John Cusack plays Brian Wilson as the very definition of a downward, depressive swing. Cusack's Wilson is burnt out, and the actor's raspy, dry and very soft voice, shaped by years of cigarette smoking, fits perfectly with Wilson at this stage of his life. My ideal version of the film, however, would cut out the Dano scenes entirely, because, as good as they are, they carry, by necessity, the air of hagiography. (The writer and director Adam Goldman created an edit of the 2009 film *Julie & Julia* – the film based on the blog by Julie Powell, in which for one year she recreated recipes by chef Julia Childs – by cutting out all of the scenes of Julie, leaving us with a perfect film about Julia Childs.)

—

For the biographical portrait of such a destructively obsessive musician, the scoring of the film needed considerable focus and fixed attention. Atticus Ross – a frequent collaborator with Trent Reznor as both a producer on Nine Inch Nails records and a co-writer of claustrophobic soundtracks for late-period David Fincher films – constructs the unique sound of *Love & Mercy* by mixing his bleak electronica with samples from Beach Boys songs, both famous and obscure. When I arrived home from New York, my second manic period began in earnest, and the soundtrack to *Love & Mercy* accompanied me, in headphones and on car stereo speakers (a rental car, again). It was some kind of sonic self-prophecy. The sound and style that Ross evokes though is true to my experience of mania, and expertly echoes the experience of both rapid speech and cyclical thought. The seven original songs almost uniformly build into crescendos, with both volume and speed increasing, as the pastiches of Brian Wilson's lyrics and dialogue pile on. This occurs most forcefully on the track 'Losing It' which appears in the film during a dinner party scene, in which the scraping of cutlery on plates grows deafeningly loud as Wilson, as played by Paul Dano, has a mealtime freak-out. The panic attack is brought on seemingly by the endless dinner party talk of his successes and future potential, and ends with Wilson begging for his guests to stop.

—

The scene reminded me immediately of one of the great moments in the catalogue of Paul Thomas Anderson films. In the 2002 film *Punch-Drunk Love*, a small business owner, Barry – played by a volatile Adam Sandler – attends a family dinner with his seven sisters and their various partners and children. On arrival, the sisters talk *at* Barry, their dialogue overlapping – incessant patter is constantly mixed into the background of the scene – and is largely made up of taunts about his sexuality ('Remember when we used to call you Gay Boy?'), which persists until Anderson cuts to a scene of Barry smashing three floor-to-ceiling windows, with both his fists and feet. If you listen closely, the scene opens with the sisters talking about Barry smashing a sliding glass door with a hammer and that 'Mum and Dad had to take him to the hospital.'

Barry pulls his brother-in-law away from the dinner, and the scene of his destructiveness, into a small laundry space, where he quietly quizzes his brother-in-law about seeking help. His brother-in-law replies, 'Barry, I'm a dentist … what kind of help do you think I can give you?'

BARRY: I'm sorry about that. I'm sorry about what I did.
WALTER THE DENTIST: It's all right.
BARRY: I wanted to ask you something because you're a doctor right. I don't like myself sometimes. Can you help me?

BARRY: Maybe you know other doctors?

WALTER THE DENTIST: Like a psychiatrist?

BARRY: I just don't have anybody else I can talk to about things. And I understand it's confidential with a doctor, and I don't want my sisters to know. I'm a bit embarrassed about this.

WALTER THE DENTIST: Barry, if it's about getting you a phone number for a psychiatrist I can do that. But what exactly is wrong?

BARRY: I don't know if there is anything wrong, because I don't know how other people are. I sometimes cry a lot … for no reason.

Barry immediately bursts into uncontrollable sobs. This outburst – alongside that deadpan dentist line – I recall being played for laughs, uncomfortable ones, at the time, but on re-watching it recently I wasn't laughing. The request for help is sincere. In the end, the brother-in-law betrays Barry's confidence, and tells his sister about his request. The family's frank discussion of his issues are increasingly frustrating through the film, and show very little signs of being well-meaning in their approach. His request is inflected with the stigma of seeking psychiatric help – fumbling, and sought in a private space – which seems contemporaneous with popular culture depictions of the time, and its ability to lend dramatic stakes. In *The Sopranos*, the foundation of the show is built on the anxiety of being exposed for seeking psychiatric assistance, a deadly reality for Tony Soprano from the first episode. It is, as ever, not clear whether these scenes are being played for laughs.

—

In a REDDIT thread, a group discusses a possible diagnosis for Barry in *Punch-Drunk Love*. They collectively go back and forth on the possibilities and how they relate:

> Seems like a pretty severe case of social anxiety and bipolar disorder causing his violent raging mood swings.

Sounds about right

> I think the anxiety disorder tendencies are spot on, however, I don't think Barry's got bipolar disorder. BPD's swings take place over a longer timeline. Ups and downs come in long waves that last months at a time.

> Barry more likely has borderline personality disorder, which is characterized by marked impulsivity (i.e. buying all that pudding, flying to Hawaii) and swings that occur at the flick of a switch. Furthermore, people with borderline personality disorder tend to view people in extremes, either holding them in very high or low esteem (i.e. his view of Lena as this perfect being).

Before a final interjection:

> Holy fucking shit that's me.

This is what cinema does to us. There is no other artform whose rate of identification runs so high. People base their morals on films. In the midst of my first mania, I walked around quoting grabs of dialogue from Daniel Plainview from *There Will Be Blood*, thinking I too was some arch and tragic figure.

—

Punch-Drunk Love was supposed to be the first film I ever saw on a date, but we missed the train to Newcastle, where we were to see it at the now defunct three-screen Show-case cinema on Wolfe Street, and so instead ended up going to see Roman Polanski's *The Pianist*. I spent the train ride home counselling my high-school girlfriend, who was dis-traught after the film, as her Polish grandparents had been survivors of the Nazi regime. I would see *Punch-Drunk Love* later on DVD. I was watching a lot of films back then and I can't remember how I felt about the movie. Anderson's work has seen some critical dissent in the last few years – many feel he is too much of a technician, and his writing leaves audiences feeling remote. His body of work is split in two, essentially, with the narrative and visual excesses of the early films (*Boogie Nights* and *Magnolia* in particular, which rush to put everything on screen) giving way to an unex-pected stateliness and classicism in *There Will Be Blood* and *The Master*. It is of note that *Punch-Drunk Love* is the film that fills this divide.

Punch-Drunk Love is not *not* a comedy. That double neg-ative is necessary because it sits in an uneasy space between its intentions and what actually appears on screen – that tension is deliberate. Anderson hasn't made a film that is explicitly about any named mental disorders, but all of his films fea-ture a character, or characters that could be broadly classified within such diagnoses: the compulsive gamblers of *Hard Eight*, the various excessive behaviours of the *Boogie Nights* cast, the increasingly strung-out ensemble of *Magnolia*, Barry in *Punch-Drunk Love*, Daniel Plainview's murderous monologue-driven rage at the end of *There Will Be Blood*, the erratic behaviour of Freddie Quell in *The Master*, and the drug-induced paranoiac air being breathed in by the low life set in *Inherent Vice*.

Magnolia is the manic depressive's movie though. It is extremely restless, and more of a music video than a film. Anderson was directing videos for his then girlfriend Fiona Apple, and the rhythm of the film comes partly from its musical sources. The influence of Scorsese carries over in this sense from *Boogie Nights* – although there are fewer pop hits used (two tracks from Supertramp's 1979 album *Breakfast in America* appear), and in their place an anxious, ever-present background theme from Jon Brion that builds and builds, with the rhythm of a ticking clock. These characters are all on a path destined to intersect; wired to burn out collectively.

In attempting to explain the sequence in which the ensemble of *Magnolia* sing along to the lyrics of Aimee Mann's 'Wise Up' towards the end of the film, the respected film scholar George Toles (a frequent collaborator with the film-maker Guy Maddin) suggests that this audacity falls in line with Anderson's approach to bringing relief to his heightened melodramatic turns:

> From the beginning of his career, Anderson has been
> drawn to operatic, bipolar contrasts between scenes of
> savage eruption and antidote scenes of containment.

What does it mean for Toles to use 'bipolar' as a critical descriptor, one that comes up fairly frequently in writing about Anderson's filmography? Metaphor manifests itself most purely in cinema, with its ability to bring together narrative, visuals and sound and so it's no coincidence that mania would be most potently expressed as allegory on screen.

—

Punch-Drunk Love is intercut with moving animations of swirling neon colours by the visual artist Jeremy Blake, a bold aesthetic choice – as ever – by Anderson. Blake was best known for obscuring the face of American indie singer-songwriter Beck for his break-up record *Sea Change*. Blake was dead by 2007; he committed suicide following the suicide of his long-time girlfriend that same year; their deaths, having occurred in such quick succession, had fascinated the media, with *Vanity Fair* even giving them a title: 'The Golden Suicides'. Bret Easton Ellis was apparently working on a film based on Blake and his girlfriend, mentioned as far back as 2009, but that has never eventuated.

Barry's storyline is marked by two impulses – one to buy pudding, the other to call a phone sex line. Anderson makes this extremely clear when he has one plot set off the other – Barry, in cutting out a coupon for the pudding, reveals underneath an advertisement for the phone service, and pushing the coupon aside with his pair of scissors, reveals the full text enticing him. This twinning – one storyline upbeat, the other decidedly down – gives the film its 'bipolar contrasts' in a narrative sense.

Barry displays other compulsive and impulsive behaviours throughout the film. He books a flight to Hawaii to visit his love interest Lena, played by Emily Watson, on a whim. And leaves her in the hospital after a car crash to travel to Utah to confront the film's villain, played explosively by Philip Seymour Hoffman. But Anderson keeps circling back to his violent outbursts.

Anderson conceived the film, in part, from a magazine article he had read in *Time*. The article told the story of The Pudding Guy – otherwise known as David Phillips – a civil engineer, who had discovered a kink in a marketing promotion run by Healthy Choice brand in 1999. Healthy Choice was offering customers the chance to earn flyer miles if they returned proof of purchase (essentially barcodes taken from the containers) of their products. The promotion, which would only last for a limited time, sent Phillips on a search for the cheapest Healthy Choice products to maximise his return on flyer miles. In searching a grocery store which moved excess products at a discount rate, he found Healthy Choice pudding cups, which sold at twenty-five cents each. Their barcode was worth the same no matter what the product, and the pudding cups were individually barcoded. Phillips went on a manic spending spree, buying 12 150 cups of pudding. He could not remove all of the barcodes in time to qualify for an early-bird special, which doubled their value, and so he enlisted the Salvation Army to help peel off the barcodes in return for donating the puddings to the charity.

The Pudding Guy had no history of mental ill health, as far as I can discover, but his spree points towards the way that late capitalism engenders behaviour that could easily be mistaken for a symptom of hypomania.

–

In the aftermath of making *Magnolia* (cancer, death, sexual abuse, dysfunction) Anderson took refuge in the films of Adam Sandler (making particular note of *Happy Gilmore* and *Big Daddy*). He also ghosted briefly on the writing staff of *Saturday Night Live*. A long-time fan of that comedy institution, during his time working within the show he directed a short film called *FANatic*, starring Ben Affleck as a die-hard fan of the troubled model and actress Anna Nicole Smith. Affleck plays Jason, who is harbouring suicidal thoughts following his parents' divorce, and through a fictitious MTV reality show called *FANatic*, he is invited to meet his famous crush. Things get stranger from there.

In an interview with Charlie Rose – with Sandler in attendance – Anderson said that it was being in a 'good mood' that led him to make *Punch-Drunk Love*. Sandler's Barry Egan – not far removed from Sandler's own stated experience of forming a self, and coming to terms with liking himself – embodied rage I have experienced. Its purity, and fear-inducing force. Sandler doesn't look like a movie star – much has been made of the fact that he provided a moment for the Jewish community to see themselves represented as the heartthrob. Sandler wasn't exactly cast against type, rather, he was cast against quality. By that, I mean simply that he hadn't done this kind of film before, nor worked with this kind of filmmaker. He had certainly used rage as a driving emotive force in his comedies *Billy Madison* and *Happy Gilmore* to great effect. That rage – with its obvious depressive qualities, both as foreshadowing and aftershocks – had also been used in a purely romantic comedy setting such as the highly effective *The Wedding Singer* (for which Carrie Fisher served as an uncredited script doctor, punching up the dialogue significantly).

—

Like *Love & Mercy*, in creating *Punch-Drunk Love* Anderson knew that sound would be just as important as any other component of the film to convey the anxious tone necessary to convey Egan's condition and inner turmoil. Working with his long-time collaborator Jon Brion (who would be replaced by Radiohead member Jonny Greenwood on his next cycle of films), to create something as disorienting as Brian Wilson's internal soundscape. If I could embed one film clip in this book it would most likely be Barry smashing a bathroom. Anderson made the decision not to re-record the sound, going with what was recorded during the film. This echoed a moment from my first manic episode: I lifted a large painting off a wall – a realistic, washed-out image of a man from the waist down, wearing faded blue jeans, painted by my mother's boyfriend from her time at art school – and threw it down the hallway. In a later episode, I took to smashing beer bottles against a wall, punching framed pictures of family members, and overturning coffee tables covered in glasses. The sound of glass breaking is the sound – for me – of the purest expression of psychic distress. To make it physical and real helps in its odd way. It's the classic 'cry for help' certainly, but it's also just the cry itself, a release.

—

Inherent Vice didn't make sense to me the first time I saw it, as it didn't for many. We walked out of the cinema in the same daze that the film's atmosphere wrapped you in. Then, in the same manic episode that took me to Canberra for Junket, it did make sense. In the Q Hotel the conference – sorry, unconference – was held in, I locked myself in my hotel room,

125

with free access to any number of recently released films, and watched the film again. Then, its paranoid edge gripped hold of me. I took selfies with the film in the background.

In a rental car (again, in Canberra), I downloaded the soundtrack, and listened compulsively to the two Jonny Greenwood songs, which featured Joanna Newsom narrating 'Spooks' (which was said to be a Radiohead demo) and 'Under the Paving-Stones, the Beach!'. 'Spooks' opens with a greeting to someone called 'Sam!'. So it was, literally, speaking to me at least.

—

Ahead of shooting *Magnolia*, Paul Thomas Anderson screened *Network* to his production team. In it, Peter Finch, in a role which would win him a posthumous Oscar, instructs a television audience that he's 'as mad as hell, and I'm not going to take this any more'. The clearer reference points for *Magnolia* were the sprawling interconnected stories of Robert Altman's cinema – namely his country music epic *Nashville* and his later adaptation of a menagerie of Raymond Carver short stories, *Short Cuts* – but Anderson takes Altman's faux-lackadaisical, carefree approach to film and tightens the grip with a more controlling, anxious direction, and a love of speed and dolly zooms and long Steadicam tracking shots lifted from Scorsese. The film feels like three hours of someone clicking their fingers at you to move faster.

Paul Thomas Anderson himself cuts a nervy figure in interview footage and the *Magnolia* documentary. Directing films requires manic energy – I don't mean to speculate on Anderson's mental health, but use the term 'manic' figuratively here, as anthropologist Emily Martin in her book

Bipolar Expeditions: Mania and Depression in American Culture references mania as a metaphor for market success and performance enhancing. Still, Anderson was using some language that would be familiar to those who have experienced mania, suggesting that his decision to make *Punch-Drunk Love* on a smaller scale was because, 'I was a madman making [*Magnolia*]. I put too much pressure on myself and I was not the person I wanted to be.'

I briefly take up smoking again, six months after quitting, after watching this short documentary – seduced by Paul Thomas Anderson's jittery smoking between moments of filming, editing or during publicity tours. This is bad, of course, but worth noting. This brief relapse occurred also on the one-year anniversary of my last manic episode, an extremely dangerous mixed-state period, in which I took up smoking as a way to do something with my hands, channel my excess of energy and steady my nerves. I quit smoking as soon as I moved back to Sydney, giving up many vices, and bad relationships, that marked my years in Melbourne.

—

The Master, released in 2012, told the story of Freddie Quell, a veteran with a likely diagnosis of PTSD. Quell has been distilled, like the alcohol he concocts out of raw found elements, to the basest instincts – sex and substance abuse. The film provided critics the purest opportunity to pathologise Quell and his mentor Lancaster Dodd (roughly based on L Ron Hubbard, the founder of Scientology) to an even greater extent than they had with Barry Egan's compulsive characteristics. Quell is the raw material for Dodd to experiment with. Two doctors test him at the start of the film – one with a series of Rorschach tests (Quell replies only in vulgar sexual terms) and one with an interview in which he is interrogated about a 'crying spell', but this is nothing compared to the interrogations to come from Dodd. The film is aware that Scientology is anti-psychiatry. Indeed, Tom Cruise surely wouldn't have worked with Anderson if *The Master* had preceded *Magnolia*. Cruise had criticised the actress Brooke Shields for her use of antidepressants in a deeply strange segment on the *Today Show* from 2005. In an interview with Matt Lauer, Cruise suggested that Shields – who had just documented her own experience of being treated for postpartum depression in her book *Down Came the Rain* – should have chosen 'vitamins and exercise' over drug therapy. Shields came at Cruise in a *New York Times* op-ed, titled 'War of Words' (punning on the film that Cruise was promoting at the time of his comments, *War of the Worlds*), writing bluntly: 'I'm going to take a wild guess and say that Mr Cruise has never suffered from postpartum depression.'

Cruise expounded on his views as his interview with Lauer took on an increasingly testy tone: 'I've never agreed with psychiatry ... ever. Before I was a Scientologist I never agreed with psychiatry. And then when I started studying the history of psychiatry I started realising more and more why I didn't agree with psychiatry. I know that psychiatry is a pseudo-science. Here we are today where I talk out against drugs and psychiatric abuses of electric shocking people against their will ...'

Lauer tried to create reason out of this mess but Cruise cut him off: 'You don't know the history of psychiatry, I do ...'

Some of that antagonistic energy would be transferred directly to Philip Seymour Hoffman's performance of

Lancaster Dodd, as a vector of L Ron Hubbard. The pseudo-science of Scientology is first and foremost hubristic arrogance. Walking around Sydney while writing this book, I discovered there was a festival dedicated to mental health happening; then, turning a corner, saw an exhibition being held in a former American Apparel storefront that led with the words: 'PSYCHIATRY IS A HUMAN RIGHTS ABUSE'. It looked grimmer than a war memorial. The stink of Scientology was in the air. I didn't dare go in, but perhaps I should have – who knows where that path would have led?

—

In the dispiriting world of academic writing, Cruise's performance as Frank TJ Mackey has been singled out as representing the emergent concept of 'bipolar masculinity'. First posited by Donna Peberdy in her book *Masculinity and Film Performance: Male Angst in Contempoary American Cinema*, and later quoted in Jason Sperb's *Blossoms and Blood: Postmodern Media Culture and the Films of Paul Thomas Anderson*, both scholars project the wild mood swings of bipolar on to forms of male acting, with Cruise, and his role in *Magnolia*, as being the exemplar. I am uneasy with non-manic depressives adopting the terminology of a serious disorder as a critical descriptor, indulging in its metaphoric qualities. (But hey, look, I'm a manic depressive so I can throw around the terminology as I see fit.) Peberdy writes, 'Rather than using "bipolar" to refer to an unstable personality disorder, I employ it here as a way of usefully describing the fluidity of both normative and non-normative constructions of masculine identity as they are enacted on the screen.' The academic language, both 'normative and non-normative', gets me down but there may be some use in looking at the demands a director like Anderson puts on a performer like Cruise. Or rather, what Anderson bottles from Cruise's inherent manic nature. But it seems no different from what is expected of Julianne Moore in the film – swinging from bravado in formal settings to a shattering breakdown in a chemist's, followed by a suicide attempt.

Peberdy suggests that the 'bipolarity' is a swing from hard to soft masculinity, which is problematic when you reapply it to its original definition. If Cruise is a hard arse in his performance of Frank TJ Mackey in this first half of the film, he is soon revealed to be hiding his true softer identity of Jack Partridge, the son of the dying television executive played by Jason Robards (Robards was dying of cancer at the time of filming his role, creating connections with real-life counterparts that touched Cruise's public vulnerabilities too). Connecting bipolarity to masculinity is strange, and the implications of tying 'soft masculinity' to emotional outbursts seems limited, and implies that hysterical performances are inherently feminine, perpetuating any number of outdated gender stereotypes. Was I feminine in the outbursts of mania – when emotions flooded over, and I screamed and 'carried on'? Are Barry Egan's problems with emotion feminine too, then? Is that why his sisters insist on calling him 'gay boy', keeping a childhood taunt going into adulthood?

—

Paul Thomas Anderson's filmography and the concept of bipolarity seem then to be eternally entwined. The critical reception of *Punch-Drunk Love* seemed to be obsessed with one particular phrase: 'a manic-depressive romantic comedy'.

It seemed to first appear in a review by the critic Charles Taylor in the online magazine *Salon*:

> *Punch-Drunk Love* is something we haven't seen before: a manic-depressive romantic comedy that aspires to the soul of a musical.

This phrasing would soon enough reappear in *Variety*:

> The shift began around the time of *Punch-Drunk Love* (2002), the manic-depressive romantic comedy starring Adam Sandler and arthouse doyenne Emily Watson. The back-to-back making of *Boogie Nights* and *Magnolia* had left Anderson feeling exhausted and eager to find a new way of working, in a looser, freer style, with a smaller crew and more room for spur-of-the-moment inspiration.

And it would later re-emerge in cinema advertisements for the film. This is from Loft Cinemas in Tucson, Arizona, which seemed to lift its copy directly from Charles Taylor's review:

> With *Punch-Drunk Love*, Paul Thomas Anderson delivers a delightfully odd and bracingly original concoction – a manic depressive romantic comedy with the soaring soul of a movie musical.

During my first mania, I broke into a bed and breakfast outside of Canberra, after my car failed on the Hume Highway. I went through the rooms of the empty lodgings and took money that was hidden through the house. I didn't really know what to do with myself or this money, so I hitched a ride into Civic Centre. I bought a ticket to see a film, but I didn't go inside the cinema. Now that I had money – more money than I needed for the moment – I wasn't quite sure what it did or what I was supposed to do with it. Why not buy a ticket to a movie without intending to actually see it? Movies did not move fast enough for me, anyway – being trapped inside a dark room, listening to someone else talk, seeing someone else's vision didn't really appeal to me when my own imagination was working in overdrive, out-Spielberging the best Hollywood directors. When I couldn't stand to be in the cinema's surrounds any longer, I walked around the shopping centre. Dead. The fatal flaws were these: it was a Sunday night and it was Canberra. This was the city where my cousin had died of an aneurism. I tried not to think about my own head.

I got back to the hotel I'd checked into earlier using the money taken from the bed and breakfast, after booking my bus ticket for the next morning. I ordered pay per view and waited up to watch *The Assassination of Jesse James by the Coward Robert Ford*, which was scheduled to screen at 2 a.m. I had seen the Andrew Dominik film in the cinema the year before and had enjoyed it. Many of the reviews I read afterwards mentioned that Jesse James, as played by Brad Pitt, was very likely a manic depressive. His erratic behaviour, in the film at least, seemed to uphold such a diagnosis. The character goes from calm in one scene, to putting a knife to a neck in the next. I wanted to see for myself if this assessment held up, but I fell asleep at the end of the first scene. No new impressions of the film were to be made that night. Things slowed down to a safer speed, but that speed was unbearable, a fact that would remain unchanged and, ironically, static for months. And it would not be the last time that a work of art would make me consider the cultural identity of the manic depressive, as it had developed and solidified across the twentieth century, and how I was to grapple with it as I came to terms with my own diagnosis.

—

I did and did not know that I was in the midst of it.

—

During this same time I terrorised many backpackers hanging around a Melbourne youth hostel with an eerie Daniel Plainview impression, repeating his iconic milkshake speech – 'I drink your milkshake, I drink it up' – over and over again verbatim. Plainview's descent into madness by film's end was one I could identify with at the time, and I wanted people to see how far gone I was.

—

In his latest film, released as I'm writing this, *Phantom Thread*, Paul Thomas Anderson crafts a story about the relationship between creative production and the small burn-outs it engenders. At the core of that process is how we rely on others to get us well. In the film, Alma, a waitress, falls for the fashion designer, Reynolds Woodcock. Their relationship seems backwards and outdated to begin with – an older man taken with a much younger woman – but soon enough Alma starts to control a wilfully difficult man, largely through poisoning him with wild mushrooms, then forcing him to rest after exhausting and demanding work periods. People mistook the film as a veneration of the male artistic temperament, but if anything it was a damnation of the man-child behaviour of the stiffly named Woodcock, and a love letter to Alma's rising power. If it buys into myths of manic creativity and the resulting depressive burn-outs, it surely does so from some place of inner truth.

—

After a hectic dress auction, Reynolds and Alma get in their car to drive to the countryside. He is clearly exhausted and she rests her hand on his temple, 'Let me drive for you.' This cuts to a scene of Reynolds in bed, which features a voice-over from a mysterious fireside interview between Alma and a doctor, who will appear, and be explained, later in the film. Alma confesses to the doctor that she likes seeing Reynolds when he is coming down from his work, partly as it shows how much he cares for the work in the first place. The doctor asks how long his 'episodes' last, and Alma replies that they only take up a few days and then Reynolds is back at work again.

—

Mania, as it manifests in cinema, is more often overly literal than not, showing the rhythms of the disorder without the reasons why. See Mike Figgis's lame *Mr Jones*, in which Richard Gere hams it up as a manic depressive, which is used to propel a romantic sub-plot, to see how wrong film can get it. Still, writing about cinema feels overly literal too – flat transcriptions of scenes.

—

If the free market and wider capitalist political economy encourage mania as a metaphor, then films too take up this cause. The ups and downs of the lives of manic depressives tend to encourage films with plots about economic distress and deception, and subsequently occupy the thriller genre. I realised this early on, just before diagnosis, say. In 2007, I went to see the newly released *Michael Clayton*, the directorial debut of Hollywood script doctor Tony Gilroy, at a cinema with a friend. We were friends because we shared issues relating to mental ill health and caught up regularly mostly just to comfort ourselves with the fact of each other's existence. This was how we connected. We also both liked drawing and had a similar taste in pop aesthetics and bright colours. *Michael Clayton* is a grim film, and from the opening scene I realised we had made a mistake in choosing it. The movie opens with a nervy, jagged narration by a character played by the British actor Tom Wilkinson. This voice-over is played over a series of shots of the dull lights of cold skyscrapers at night and their empty office spaces. It has a purposefully claustrophobic effect. Wilkinson's character is leaving a phone message for the titular character, Michael Clayton:

> All I'm saying is wait, just wait, just … just, just please
> hear me out. Because this is not an episode, relapse,
> fuck up. I'm begging you Michael, I'm begging you
> … try and make believe that this is not just madness,
> because this is not just madness.

This narration sets up the paranoid tone of the film and the plot turns to come. My friend was clearly not enjoying this start to the film and, leaning over, whispered that she was going to leave the cinema and meet me later in the food court. I stayed, because I was transfixed by Wilkinson's character and how those around him treated him. How did mania seem to outsiders? Could this movie show people just how fast someone in the midst of it can talk? Rapid speech, after all, is one of mania and hypomania's most vexing symptoms.

—

In 2009, Steven Soderbergh, working with one of his preferred screenwriters Scott Z Burns, adapted a nonfiction book based on the career and life of scientist Mark Whitacre, called *The Informant!* That exclamation mark in the title seems key to the whole premise, going some way to pointing to the energy of the film, and Whitacre's larger-than-life mishaps. Matt Damon played Whitacre as a white-collar criminal, who first informed the FBI of price-fixing within his company, and by his associates, before embezzling funds from the same company himself. Damon provides a flat, distracted voice-over for his character, which runs through the entire film, speculating on off-hand thoughts as Whitacre divulges trade secrets to entrusted law enforcers. His mind wanders. Whitacre's diagnosis with bipolar disorder, ultimately, had little sway over the judge overseeing his case and he served eight and a half years in a federal prison.

Soderbergh plays with his usual palette of saturated colours here – seen to great, dissociative effect in earlier films, where warm oranges similarly dominate – but he also introduces and pushes the lighting to a sense of overexposure, which gives the film a certain fuzziness. Part of this works to make the film feel like a 1970s jaunt, but it also provides a washed-out feeling – an uneasy haze – that stands in line with Whitacre's blurry logic and cumulative lies. Soderbergh would go on to make the pharmaceutical thriller *Side Effects*, which parodied some of the tropes of contemporary psychiatry to craft a campy B movie.

Damon buzzes along but doesn't play it full loon, possibly because the diagnosis had to be hidden for narrative purposes.

—

My wife and I saw one of the best of these films about manic-depression at the end of our time in New York that fateful year. On the day before our return flight home, we were sitting in the Sunshine Cinema in the lower east side of Manhattan, holding tickets to see the comedy *Infinitely Polar Bear*. The film's clunky name is the worst title imaginable, one that actively repels, but we had come for its depiction of manic-depressive illness. I was well enough, having survived the tumult of New York City for the most part. And the trip home was promising. We sat up the back and eased into our seats. A midday screening was all we had time for and the cinema was empty. The film was written and directed by Maya Forbes, who had previously worked as a screenwriter and TV producer for *The Larry Sanders Show*. Forbes wrote the film on the insistence of Wes Anderson, who was dating Forbes' sister at the time, after meeting her father, Cameron Forbes. As a group they had taken her father out to lunch, breaking him out of his temporary home at McLean, the infamous psychiatric hospital near Boston. On returning him, Cam, as he was affectionately called, came running outside with two cigarettes in his mouth. Anderson would use that image for Bill Murray's listless character in his break-out film *Rushmore* (a kind of despondent, 'got no fucks to give' look that I obsessed over while falling in love with that film as a teenager). But Forbes got the bulk of the material, having grown up with an increasingly eccentric father-on-the-fringe. Cam Forbes becomes Cam Stuart in the film, but the details hew close to life, with Maya Forbes' daughter – Imogene Wolodarsky – playing a younger version of her mother.

Cam's struggles with manic depression meant that he had been kicked out of both Harvard and Exeter, 'for very different reasons', and met his wife working in public television, but is unemployed by the time the film begins. Mark Ruffalo – the charm-to-spare Hollywood hunk – plays a very fit looking Cam. Maybe all that nervous energy lays waste to body fat.

The most noteworthy aspect of the film goes further than its depiction of Cam's manic depressive episodes; it is in its exploration of the responsibility of work, and the division of labour within a family unit when someone is diagnosed with an ongoing psychiatric disorder. What is that person capable of, and what is the breaking point? The film largely focuses on the decision that Cam will look after his two young daughters while his wife, Maggie, from whom he is separated, goes on to study towards an MBA in New York. Economic realities have hit the family – Cam's family are from a wealthy background, but the wealth is not shared, and must be begged for in front of a controlling grandmother. There are the realities of economic disparity for those who cannot work due to their condition. His wife knows how his condition blocks him from making money: 'And he had a job which was really good for him. He was a terrific lighting designer. But in the end it was too much pressure for him. And I didn't know ... I didn't know about manic-depression, besides it was the 60s. Everyone was having nervous breakdowns.'

She warns him to see his privilege in the situation: 'When white people live in squalor, they're eccentric. When black people live in squalor, no one is charmed ... believe me.'

The only physical violence he displays is in fighting for his wife to get a job at a business firm related to his family. Afterwards, he comes home and immediately takes his lithium medication.

The film deals responsibly and directly with the realities of parenthood, particularly fatherhood, when living with manic depression. This is something I have given a lot of thought to when considering having children. Cam lives with his diagnosis while parenting two young children with great bravery and sacrifice to serve them as best as he can. He falters, and he fails: he gives up one night, heading out to a bar for a night of clear excess. He hoards. Despite this he is, undoubtedly, good with kids: from cooking to other general domestic duties, documented throughout the film. The building they live in is filled with single mothers – Cam is jealous of them meeting up for coffee, and having wine and cheese nights. 'They never invite me,' he laments. One tenant commends him, albeit backhandedly: 'I just have to say my ex-husband would never do what you're doing, I think it's so evolved. Most men would be completely emasculated by having their wife go off to be the bread winner'.

When we left the film we sat in a branch of Whole Foods, eating tubs of salad, near the cinema. Outside there was a mural of the Hulk – played by a digitised version of Ruffalo in various incarnations in the unstoppable Marvel film franchise – visible from our seats and it would be the last image of this particular American journey. Looking out onto it as we waited for a taxi to take us to the airport, I wondered about all these depictions of manic depression on screen. At the end of the film, when it is decided that Maggie will take the children to live with her in New York, Cam speculates: 'I can't visit you in New York. Too much speed and noise and all the people on the streets all night … it knocks me off track.' It turned out I could visit New York, but not for too long. The city carries within it an infinite number of triggers for mania (staggering down Times Square, walking alone, and drunk, perhaps I had tipped into that space). Occasionally, as a compulsive film completist, I feel the same way about cinema. But I simply couldn't make sense of my life without it.

6

UNDER HER INFLUENCE

An imagined audio commentary for John Cassavetes' *A Woman Under the Influence* (1974) between Sam Twyford-Moore and the fictitious film scholar and psychologist FSP.

FSP: Is it synced up? Are we synced up with the movie? Do we need to start again? I don't think we'll talk about every scene, right, just intercut between the important parts?

STM: Yeah, I think that's how we will do it. We don't have to be precise about the timing, people will watch the film in their own way. It's a long movie. About two hours and twenty minutes – all of Cassavetes' movies ran to something like that. They could all probably have about half an hour cut from them without missing much, but that's just a personal opinion. Anyway, we're transcribing this for the book, so it won't be actual audio, so people will have to find the parts of the movie we are talking about on their own time.

FSP: Could we release the audio though?

STM: Possibly, I'd have to ask the publishers about that.

FSP: Can you tell us why you wanted to talk about this film in particular?

STM: This is the complete picture of a reckoning with mania, and manic depression, that we were talking about throughout this book, and that picture is available on import as a Criterion Collection DVD. Watching Gena Rowlands in *A Woman Under the Influence*, in a mid-film climactic breakdown, pacing back and forth, hands twitching, trying to count towards something – anything – I held my breath for what felt like minutes. I could see myself in that portrayal – the confusion as to personal loyalties when people are just trying to care for you and make sure you get well; the counterintuitive belief in conspiracies during this period. Paranoia grips and does not let go, and sabotages the one thing that will get you through.

FSP: Where are we at? About five minutes in?

STM: Yeah. We first see Mabel Longhetti, barefoot, in her front yard, trying to help organise her kids to go off with their grandmother. She's pretty erratic in that introduction. But nothing seems off, necessarily. The grandmother does say, 'Your mother is terribly nervous' though.

FSP: Nervous seems the right word for it, right?

STM: Yeah, I like nervous a lot – as in nervous breakdown, because it really does relate to the nerves. It seems like a bit old-fashioned now, like manic depressive I guess, but it's still true, right?

FSP: She talks to herself a lot in that scene – a sign of things to come?

STM: I guess so; it's an interesting intro. She bops around to some opera too.

FSP: So yeah, but it's John Cassavetes directing, yeah? Have we said that yet?

STM: Yeah. He directs. Apparently he originally wrote the film as a play, but realised that he couldn't ask an actress to play Mabel eight times a week. It would just be too tough to inhabit that character, and all her moods and breakdowns, at that length. It is an extremely demanding role, and a lot is asked of Gena Rowlands.

FSP: Rowlands was Cassavetes' wife. Do you think he could have asked someone else to play the role?

STM: Absolutely not. No matter what Cassavetes' intentions were – scripting and direction and the rest – it all comes down to Gena Rowland's embodiment of Mabel Long-hetti. Throughout their collaborations, Rowland carried whichever film she appeared in.

FSP: What is the basic story?

STM: Well, on the basic scale, it's the story of Mabel, a house-wife, and her husband, Nick, a construction worker, as they deal with her breakdown, hospitalisation and for the final part, her recovery.

FSP: So where are we in the film now?

STM: Okay, we are almost in the bar scene … Mabel has had a six pack of beer, and some cigarettes, and has her feet up on the table. She's kind of deciding to go out, I guess. This is about like what, ten minutes in? The thing that people tend to forget is that Mabel sleeps around, she cheats on her husband, and I do wonder if this has some-thing to do with the sexual promiscuity that comes about from mania. Here she is picking up this dropkick in a bar, and bringing him back to the family home, knowing that Nicky will be home in the morning sometime. It's extremely audacious on her part. The indiscretion won't be so secret for long, not like this.

FSP: According to Wikipedia, Cassavetes wrote the film for Rowlands, but as a play, to deal with the difficulties experienced by contemporary women. That's an under-statement! What makes her performance, what makes it an embodiment of mania, for you?

STM: It's all in the way that Rowlands' face twitches, the way it turns, and appears to chew itself from inside. She's computing her feelings in real time – she knows something isn't right with her mind, and she expresses that in the most incredible way. It's difficult to get that right, to externalise a complex set of emotions, but it's true to the experience for me. You are confused, and lost and bewildered. That requires a deeply expressive face.

FSP: What else do you like about the movie?

STM: Cassavetes' formlessness – his drift – fits the narrative of breakdown and recovery almost perfectly. The return from the brink is as important as the edge, and the act of falling over it, itself. What Cassavetes gets right about mania is the musicality and its rhythm of its restlessness. In a montage early in the film, the main character played by Gena Rowlands can't sit still. It becomes apparent that she is internally debating whether or not to go out for more drink. Empty blue beer cans are strewn around her.

FSP: Nick seems like a sweet soul – a devoted husband for sure. Is it a romance?

STM: He stands by her. He really does. I guess it's a romantic film, it's not a comedy, not a romantic comedy. I'm not sure what it is exactly. But it is definitely love, pure and true. Nick comes to her defence, talking to a colleague: 'Mabel's not crazy. She's unusual, she's not crazy, so don't say she's crazy. This woman cooks, sews, makes the bed, cleans up the bedroom, what the hell is crazy about that?'

FSP: Okay, we're up to the scene where Mabel makes dinner

for Nick and his work colleagues – a big communal dinner of spaghetti, and talk is … weird, it has a very distinct style in this scene.

STM: The family dinner table is a place of concentrated extremes of social etiquette – taking a seat is practically signing a social contract of manners and ways of behaving – so it is unsurprising that filmmakers find it inviting as the spot for climactic breakdowns and odd, out-of-sync behaviours.

FSP: What do you think of Cassavetes as an actor, he's not in this, but I can't help but think of him – is he kind of acting through his camera movements, does that make sense?

STM: They're fine – he is a very close cameraman. You can see set photographs of him with the camera right up in the faces of the actors.

FSP: Okay, we're at the big centrepiece scene – Mabel is confronted by a doctor, her husband and her awful, awful mother-in-law.

STM: One thinks that it could all turn out like *Rosemary's Baby* at any moment, which, funnily enough, starred Cassavetes as the scheming husband to Mia Farrow's Rosemary. The scales could tip at any moment revealing a massive familial conspiracy to medicate Mabel into pure stupor. Everyone – and I mean everyone – around her is acting crazy. They don't know how to contain her, so they go a little mad themselves. They carry on, and they go large. Nicky is distraught, and his mother – Mabel's mother-in-law – wants to project her influence, and to project is really to pitch your performance, and your voice by the way, at a volume that is louder than the person you're talking to

– really to put them into submission. So, she goes large. And it's an odd performance from that actress. How do you possibly respond to Rowlands in that heightened state? How do you reach out to her? Well, you have to get hysterical, a little hysterical. You have to match her somehow, to somehow meet her at her level. The film is kind of deafening like that. Nothing flattens out though – I think that's important, nothing, and I mean nothing, flattens out.

FSP: God, Cassavetes just gets the madness right.

STM: Is it any wonder that a documentary on Cassavetes making *Love Streams* – basically his final film – is called *I'm Almost Not Crazy*? I could say the same for myself, but I am, at some molecular level, very crazy indeed. Perhaps crazy isn't the right word – crazed is probably more precise.

FSP: Does all this, then, carry a personal meaning for you?

STM: I met a friend recently for an early morning coffee in a relaxed Sydney café. She was running late. I didn't care. She asked me to meet her to talk about her recent diagnosis and hospitalisation. I had been in her home months before and she had had a vintage poster for *A Woman Under the Influence* hanging, framed, on the wall. The seeds were there for this kind of identification with Mabel and her distress. And it's not to suggest some premeditation nor falsity, just that we seek out the culture before we seek out the diagnosis and before we know the truth. We are all, somehow, under her influence.

FSP: This movie is long.

STM: I'm sort of at the point where I would prefer to watch any other Cassavetes movie. This is too much heartbreak to bear, but also I've just thought about this film for too long. It lives in my system somewhere, and I don't actually need to watch it for that reason. Turn it off. I said turn it fucking off. Are you listening to me, turn it off you motherfucker.

WAYS
OF
BEING

7

SPEAK, SPALDING!

I used to have a mortifying habit of impersonating figures from films for days, sometimes weeks, on end. Somewhere I had read about Peter Sellers feeling that he didn't
have an actual sense of self – that he was always acting as
either one of his creations, or his creation of 'Peter Sellers'. I decided that, yes, this was true for me too; except
I had no talent for creating fictitious characters, so I just
adopted other people's. Any number of Robin Williams or
Jim Carrey or Adam Sandler roles – any variation on the
man-child comics who had obsessed me at fourteen or so
– gave me tics and accents to work with. I had a particular gift for walking around for hours talking like screaming celebrity chefs. I adopted the sheepish walk and nervy
manner of Anthony Perkins in *Psycho* for a few weeks. It
was like being in a perpetual state of method acting without a job to slip into at the end of it to excuse the over-
bearingness. It easily tipped from being a twenty-second
impression in front of friends to a two-week, lived-in
performance piece. I might as well have rented a theatre.
The worst came when I spent a week talking like Robert
Crumb after seeing Terry Zwigoff's humiliating eponymous documentary, *Crumb*, about the legendary cartoonist.
Then again, at least I didn't do an impression of one of his

brothers; Maxon and Charles Jnr Crumb both succumbed to darker depths of disorder than their middle brother.

Still, who knows what other people thought of this, or if any of them had seen the documentary. I recall subjecting one poor classmate to a two-hour encore of this performance on the slow train ride from Sydney towards Newcastle. I was still glued to this Crumb impression, and so, in some bizarre attempt to impress my classmate, subjected him to the nervy voice of the weirdo comic artist who, as the Australian art critic Robert Hughes suggests in Zwigoff's documentary, is 'basically the Bruegel of the last half of the twentieth century'.

This poor guy got off the train right before the Hawkesbury River and I sincerely hope he didn't throw himself into the water. As for me, thankfully I shook off that ugly Crumb impression soon enough, and with the shame of that train ride in my mind, and as I began to feel fully myself, shook off the habit too. We learn by mimicking others, but at a certain point you've got to go it alone. This desire to be someone else – did it come from having a mood disorder, which might have led to a scattered personality and sense of self? Or did it come from being a writer, someone who reads to understand others and writes in order to be others – except that I've ended up writing mostly about myself. The drive towards obsessive autobiographical writing and observation is nothing new.

⎯

In her restless novel *Sleepless Nights*, Elizabeth Hardwick quotes a question posed, originally, by Jorge Luis Borges: 'Are not the fervent Shakespeareans who give themselves over to a line of Shakespeare, are they not, literally, Shakespeare?'

⎯

Does mania invite mimicry? Don't we all want to act outrageously every now and then? In her collage-like novel *Speedboat* Renata Adler relates a story – true or untrue; the trick of reading that novel is to go between what is real and what is fiction, and to let each seep in together – of the French singer Edith Piaf. The artist was performing her last concerts at the Paris Olympia. She sings 'Je ne suis pas folle' and 'ended the song, as always, with maniac laughter'. Adler, as her narrator-self, continues: 'On this particular evening, someone way back in the theater echoed that laughter. At first, it was thought to be a prankster, or at least a heckler. Then it was thought to be part of the performance. But when that insane laugh continued, bitter, chilling, on Edith Piaf's precise note, like one tuning fork of madness responding to another, three ushers and six members of the audience escorted the laughing lady, with infinite courtesy, to the street.'

—

Touring Australia in 1948 with her husband, Laurence Olivier, and the Old Vic Company, Vivien Leigh experienced bouts of mania. The entire troupe was aware of this, and according to Michelangelo Capua's biography of her, they mimicked her actions in order to make her appear sane, or otherwise appease her. Leigh would remove her jewellery and fussily order it, which was seen by many as the first sign of a manic episode. The actors soon enough began to do the same – taking off jewellery, ordering it, cleaning it obsessively – whenever she started this process. This is a strange intervention. I wonder what the mark of the beginning of a manic episode would be like for me, and what it would look like if my friends came together and started mimicking my behaviour.

I would probably be deeply disturbed and pissed off at them, and tell them to fuck off.

—

Sometimes you find the person who is the closest possible approximation to yourself you can imagine, and you both want to be them, and don't want to be them. Watching the late Jonathan Demme's *Swimming to Cambodia* on dodgy YouTube uploads, I saw the figure of the person I thought I really was: the actor and monologuist Spalding Gray. Yet there was no way I could impersonate him. This was because Spalding Gray was, first and foremost, himself. This isn't the same as saying that he was self-confident or self-content – most of his monologues counter just this – but you can't say that he was *not* himself. Which is likely derived from his ability to express these very anxieties, and refined by his obsession with autobiographical storytelling. If you repeat stories of the self, do you not become more yourself with each telling? And then the question becomes this: does that make you more, or less, out of the reach of impersonation? I was less my self than Spalding Gray was his self. This can certainly be true of people; think of the expression 'he was fully in his own skin'. The opposite is a state of being barely in one's own skin.

I was thinking all of this because I was thinking about the self and how it gets made, and it was clear that part of this came from impersonation – performance – and I wonder if that's because I was *nuts*. In David O Russell's underrated and determinedly anarchic comedy *I Heart Huckabees*, a central pseudo-philosophical question arises when the straitlaced character, played by Jude Law, asks, 'How am I not myself?' Dustin Hoffman and his fellow 'existential detective', played by Lily Tomlin, who are interviewing Law's character as part of their 'case', become enamoured with the phrasing and repeat it over and over again, as if trying to unpack its meaning by altering the pronunciation slightly with each repetition.

—

'How am I not myself?' 'How am I not myself?'

—

One of the many, many horrors of depression is that it takes your words away from you. You realise the other person is talking, and you haven't been saying anything for hours on end. This is a painful inversion of mania's excess of speech. You simply run out of words at some point. This is what they mean by the two poles of 'bipolar'. I remember sitting in a bar in early December one year, realising that depression had taken hold at last, and wanting to be able to speak, to offer something – but nothing came. I painfully sat through nights like this all that summer, wishing to be dead. I would sit at parties, across from semi-strangers, just staring into my beer, terrified to talk, terrified of talk. The summer before I hadn't been able to stop. People were in my court, then – now, not so much. As if I had run dry, and felt it – a cruel feeling. The pit of my stomach felt empty. An inability to pull anything up and out to put on offer. The problem was my job at the time required much talk – it was all board meetings, stakeholder engagement and artist liaison. In a meeting with a major sponsor, I could find nothing to say. A colleague came out of the meeting, and commented, 'Sorry if I talked too much.' I wanted to reply, 'No, you saved me, thank you.' The work was social, built from engaging with people. If only I were a people person, I cried. Well, I had been once, but I had spent my social capital.

—

What would it have been like for Gray, at the end of his life, robbed of language, when his very livelihood relied on words for its very construction? It pains me to think of his pain. Driving in Ireland in 2001 – on a holiday celebrating his sixtieth birthday – Gray, travelling without a seatbelt in the backseat of the car, was knocked unconscious after a collision with a veterinarian's van. Gray knocked his head against that of his wife, Karen Russo. While Russo sustained minor injuries, Gray awoke with permanent damage. The recovery would be long, and torturous. And, in a critical way, he never did truly recover, his depression taking a death-grip.

Gray consulted with the neurologist and writer Oliver Sacks, and his colleague Orrin Devinsky, two years after his accident. In a long essay for the *New Yorker* – 'The Catastrophe: Spalding Gray's Brain Injury' – Sacks outlined his treatment of Gray in the last years of his life. It was a slow process of returning Gray to wellness, and also to his writing. Gray had become fixated on what he believed to have been the horrific mistake of selling his house. Sacks writes that Gray 'later came to feel that he was "not himself" at the time, that "witches, ghosts, and voodoo" had "commanded" him to do it'. Sacks covers Gray's history with psychological problems, and various diagnoses:

> Spalding had had occasional depressions, he said, for more than twenty years, and some of his physicians thought that he had a bipolar disorder. But these depressions, though severe, had yielded to talk therapy, or, sometimes, to treatment with lithium.

This time something was different. According to Sacks, '[Gray] tried to converse with others, especially his children, but found it difficult. His ten-year-old son and his sixteen-year-old stepdaughter were distressed, feeling that their father had been "transformed" and was "no longer himself".'

—

In 2002, following his car accident, Gray voluntarily admitted himself to a psychiatric hospital, but did so using a pseudonym: Mr Edward Jones. It is hard to understand why, exactly. Gray was not the kind of famous where such an admission would be reported upon, and it seems unlikely that any colleagues, friends or close relations who he didn't want to find out would have been closely examining this hospital's admissions list. Perhaps it goes back to the point that during states of mania, or even melancholia, the sense of self is entirely removed.

—

When asked, at an event at New York's IFC Center honouring the anniversary of *Swimming to Cambodia*, if Spalding spoke at the same rapid pace of his monologues, his ex-wife Renée Shafransky replied: 'He wasn't working that way in his head all the time. And that said, eight shows a week, doing that, can get the chemicals imbalanced, and he had some of that. He was diagnosed with some bipolar and I spent six months with him when he was on lithium and that was as long as he would take it for. It was like being with a completely different person and I could understand why he did not want to continue with that.'

—

Reading his *New York Times* obituary, I find that they say he practised the art of storytelling with a 'quiet mania'. I don't quite get the idea of 'quiet mania'. The *New York Times* is right to invoke volume, however. Gray's mastery is part volume control – and that is, in a way, a modulation of his self. Big and small, loud and quiet. Are these not operatic, bipolar swings too? On a particularly electric New Year's Eve, I end up having a couple of friends on the manic spectrum over, neither of whom had met each other, and part of the guessing and waiting game of the party ahead was wondering who would silence who. It was uncomfortable to watch this big personality wrestling match, and when someone seemed to have 'won', the other went into quiet introspection – uncertain terrain for the loud and boisterous. I would like to never host another party like that again.

—

How am I not myself? Self-awareness is intolerable in its own way, and new knowledge can be crippling and extremely dangerous. Gray's mother seemed to have encountered this problem. In his autobiographical novel *Impossible Vacation* – commissioned and written after the success of his mono- logues, and seeming to take in much of the same material, to the point that the novel can only be read with Gray's voice in mind – Gray takes his mother to see the filmic adaptation of *Who's Afraid of Virginia Woolf?*.

'I made a big mistake', he writes. Gray's mother over- identifies with the role of Martha, played by Elizabeth Taylor, and tells her husband the next morning that she thinks she might *be* Martha. Gray's mother – or is it Martha, now? – wanted to see the Mike Nichols–directed adaptation because she had become fascinated by the death of Virginia Woolf; the original play, of course, never mentions the famous writer in any way.

> She wanted to go because she had this fascination with
> the life and death of Virginia Woolf. I'm not sure that
> she knew Virginia Woolf's books all that well, but she
> did know the story of how Woolf ended her life by
> filling her pockets with rocks and walking into a river.
> She seemed to know that story as well as the story of
> how Hart Crane, depressed one morning, walked off
> the stern of his cruise ship in the Gulf of Mexico, never
> to be seen again.

This creates a chilly echo, given Spalding's eventual form of suicide. I came to the work of Spalding Gray following his death. I had the exact details in mind as I discovered the mono- logues. A long, loving profile, 'Vanishing Act', published by *New York* magazine and searchable online, detailed Gray's disappearance in January 2004. His family last saw him after he took his children to see Tim Burton's *Big Fish*, the story of a son reckoning with his dying father and his past. Gray's body would be discovered two months later, surfacing on the East River. He had jumped off the Staten Island Ferry. The boat's staff had seen him on the ferry just days before he disappeared, and had made note of the figure, after he had left his wallet on a seat and walked to the edge of the vessel. In that instance, security guards accompanied Gray off the boat. He left no suicide note, which had confused his family. It signalled that he was truly lost for words.

An interest in public figures due to their circumstances of death is an unhealthy obsession. It is literally a dead end.

—

Spalding Gray became himself under uneasy circumstances. He was born in 1941 and raised in Barrington, Rhode Island, the middle child of three boys. His mother was a strict Christian Scientist, and committed suicide while he was in his mid twenties. His early life was marked by her frequent depressions, and her refusal to seek treatment due to her religion. He lived closely against the grain of this genetic connection to madness and often ruminated on his inheritances from his mother – the anxiety and depression. For many, this genetic trace is kept at a generation's remove, but for Gray it was very close indeed. It is among the first questions they ask in the diagnostic phase: 'Have you had a family member who was known to suffer from this or that condition?'

—

Gray came up in acting through The Performance Group – an experimental theatre troupe established by Richard

Schechner in 1967 – performing and co-writing on several collaborative works in New York City. *Commune* – a group work whose sole sustained scene depicted the murder of Sharon Tate, echoing Joan Didion's obsession in *The White Album* – was made up largely of quotations, a collage-like piece of contemporary theatre. Gray joined a workshop led by the actress Joyce Aaron, in which one of the primary exercises was simply standing and telling your own story based on your experience from that day. Gray excelled in this form and would later reflect on this process as creating a 'memory film', in which he had no trouble editing whatever material he chose *as* he spoke. The talent was clear, then. A trilogy of performances with The Wooster Group – a new collective originating in 1975 with works written and directed by Gray and Elizabeth LeCompte – would follow Gray's 'autobiographical impulses' into an exploration of the development of the self in relation to language. The first, *Sakonnet Point* (1975), was a 'silent mood piece which represented the child before speech' and the second, *Rumstick Road* (1977) 'was about the child learning to speak by listening and imitating'. Footage of Gray performing *Sakonnet Point* has survived online. In the short video extract Gray plays with a model plane, his body incredibly lean, and his only vocal, a long whine to emulate the plane taking off. He is without speech – primal and childlike – and this clear understanding of the role that language plays in forming identity would lead Gray to his breakthroughs in the monologue form. The third and final work, *Nayatt School* (1978), in what would become known as *Three Places in Rhode Island*, would take him even closer to his destined artform. The play, a deconstruction of TS Eliot's *The Cocktail Party*, opened with a short monologue about Gray's relationship to Eliot's work, and featured an early prototype of his delivery, seated, at a wooden table. It is important to note that this formlessness and experimentation leads into a more 'straightforward' form of storytelling. This movement is a kind of literary journeying. Gray's monologues were radical in their reductions, but they could only be what they were because of the restlessness of 'Spalding Gray', and the way he succumbed to it. That restlessness was inherent to both his artistic pursuit, and his innate character. The American poet Carl Phillips explores such notions and points of connections in depth in his essay, 'On Restlessness':

> ... there is a sensibility that – instinctively, most likely unconsciously – recognizes vulnerability as a zone of possible illumination. For such a sensibility, the impulse is not to shun the unknown but to offer the self up to it, for the chance to know the self more completely than before: for at least one way in which we come to know ourselves comes from observing how we succeed or do not succeed in meeting any given challenge.

Phillips also contends: 'Another way to think of restlessness: as a form of ambition.' Gray certainly used it that way, as do many artists, as do many who experience mania. In 1979, he debuted *Sex and Death to the Age 14*, the first of his longform, standalone monologues and one that signalled both his autobiographical drive and how much of himself he was going to hand over to the audience. In an interview nearly a decade later, David Letterman asked, 'How did this begin?' Gray mentioned his training with The Performance Group, before diverting to something both more comic and more truthful:

'I was talking a lot. I wanted to go into therapy. I thought I could talk it out there. Classical psychoanalysis. But they rejected me three times at the Columbia Presbyterian Institute.'

'Oh, why?' Letterman drolly continues.

'Oh, they said I travel too much and that real deep therapy was a very dangerous thing and that I should go into mild therapy first – you know, one hour a week – but I wanted to talk every night, or every day, so I started doing it to my audience.'

Gray walked out onto the set of the *Late Show with David Letterman* confident. Letterman quizzed him about what to call him. Gray pulled a piece of paper from the back pocket of his pants, and offered a counter: 'So today I was going through trying to figure out who I was exactly … I ate half a pound of turkey which has a natural enzyme in it – tryptophan – which … ' 'Helps you relax', Letterman adds. Then Gray lists a set of alternatives for describing Spalding Gray:

A WASP Woody Allen based on Norman Rockwell
A combination of Russell Baker and Mr Rogers
Ralph Lauren playing a younger version of Carl
    Sandburg
A combination of Huck Finn and Candide
A horny pilgrim
A new-wave version of Mark Twain
A male Lily Tomlin
An intricate trick box
A cross between David Letterman and Andy Warhol

David Letterman goes for that last option: 'There you go, that's the one.' So, Spalding Gray, being interviewed by David

Letterman, is half David Letterman. Gray doesn't have Letterman's trademark cynicism in that interview; again, he is softly spoken but that acerbic wit, and the very causticity of it, could be seen in moments of the monologues. It was never quite anger in the monologues, which is astonishing given his entire body of work seemingly stems from the injustice of losing his mother, and inheriting her nervous disposition.

—

The audience is tricked into thinking there is something spontaneous about the performance, but it is carefully crafted. In one early monologue, however, Gray responded to prompts taken randomly from a box of cards. There were spontaneous imperfections; he stumbled over words, but anyone would, talking that fast. And the imperfections are their own form of perfection – an admission and embodiment of vulnerability is necessary to win over the audience.

From his diary: 'We crave an increasingly intimate relationship with the author, unmediated, in so far as possible, by the contrivance of art'. A curious reversal takes place. The finished works serve as a prologue to the jottings; the published book becomes a stage to be passed through – a draft – en route to the definitive pleasure of the notes, the fleeting impressions, the sketches in which it had its origins.

—

Swimming to Cambodia was released in American cinemas in 1987 and almost immediately changed the trajectory of Spalding's career. It would no longer be a one-man show exactly, as there were now collaborators from the world of film knocking on his door. The first was Jonathan Demme – off the back of his energetic road caper *Something Wild*, and a few years out from his own mainstream success with *The Silence of the Lambs* – who had Gray cut down the two parts of *Swimming to Cambodia* into a single whole and brought his own visual vocabulary to the project. He intensified Gray's neurotic patter. He had done something similar for David Byrne's nervy movements in the Talking Heads concert film *Stop Making Sense*. Demme is best known for the extreme lengths to which he pursues a subjective camera point of view: the actor or performer delivers their lines straight into the lens, creating a near-claustrophobic intimacy.

Demme came to the project at the invitation of Gray's wife Renée Shafransky and was excited by its potential. He had noted that Louis Malle's *My Dinner with Andre* had been an unexpected success, and it got him thinking that if a non-fiction-ish documentary about two people talking could be successful, why not a documentary of just one person speaking? Demme, after all, understood Gray's perfect modulation of a single voice – softly spoken in the right moment, booming only occasionally, usually as Gray's excitement, and pressured speech, ramps up – and just a hint of a gentle, disarming lisp. (A lisp, how I long for a lisp! I think a lisp can make someone sound infinitely smarter.) Jonathan Demme picks up on this more than any other director of Gray's screen adaptations – zooming in and dimming the lights at just the right points to focus you in on this perfect habit of Gray's, his ability to direct your attention intensely. Laurie Anderson's confident, bass-heavy score – perfectly of its time – underlines all this.

Gray exposes the fragility of fictions – particularly ones set overseas and during wartime. These recreations tend to break people's minds. Asia, too, is known for testing the tourists' mental limits. Francis Ford Coppola lost his mind on the Philippines set of *Apocalypse Now*, as documented in *Hearts of Darkness*. On the set of that film, it wasn't just Coppola: Dennis Hopper, Marlon Brando and Martin Sheen all represented a kind of madness too.

—

Gray's generative capacity became clear as his body of work grew. The books became, increasingly, about the preceding works. *Monster in a Box*, for example, directly refers to the writing of the novel *Impossible Vacation* in its title – the novel is the monster that haunts Spalding. The novel isn't his best work – it mimics the form of the monologues, reciting incidents, but doesn't have the character of his inflections – but then he wasn't ever supposed to be a novelist. *Monster in a Box* resulted regardless, springing with new life from the frustrations of the novel-writing process, and might be the best of the many monologues. It is largely about his manuscript for *Impossible Vacation* as it spirals to become 1400 pages long. During this period, he took a trip to Russia with a number of famous writers and artists, touring the film version of *Swimming to Cambodia*. Carrie Fisher was on the tour, and I would give a kidney to eavesdrop on the conversations between these two famous manic depressives. She is only mentioned when Gray boards a tour bus organised for the performers on a day off. He writes/speaks a comic stretch about a domino effect of the stars getting on and off the bus, delaying its departure:

> Renée and I got on at ten o'clock. Ten-thirty, Carrie
> Fisher gets on. She looks around, she doesn't see

anyone. She gets off and writes another chapter of her book. Daryl Hannah gets on the bus. She doesn't see Carrie Fisher. Daryl Hannah gets off and searches for coffee with caffeine. Marlee Matlin doesn't see Daryl Hannah, doesn't see Carrie Fisher. ... Richard Gere gets on the bus. Richard Gere looks around, doesn't see Carrie Fisher, doesn't see Daryl Hannah, doesn't see Marlee Matlin, doesn't see Matt Dillon. Richard gets off the bus and goes and writes a letter to the Dalai Lama.

—

In *Impossible Vacation*, the big break for Spalding's alter-ego Brewster – and, in truth, Spalding Gray himself – came when he starred in a play written by another manic depressive, Robert Lowell. Gray wrote in the voice of Brewster, 'I loved Robert Lowell at a distance. I didn't want to get too close because he represented that New England over-breeding which led to hypersensitivity and periodic madness, as well as wicked bouts with alcohol. He was a noble, beautiful man to look at, but deep in his writing I could feel him like an overbred Irish setter; nervous, quivering and shaking, constantly on the edge.'

—

Gray eventually came to categorise his growing body of work as 'autofiction'. He lived it as he wrote it. In the *Terrors of Pleasure* – a work concerned mostly with Gray hunting for the perfect property – exasperated, he cries, 'Did I buy this piece of shit house just to write a monologue about it?' In the same monologue, he consults self-help books during a particularly panicked period. I consult Spalding Gray when I'm nervous and in need of help, his help.

—

Is it any surprise that when the filmmaker Steven Soderbergh came to make a documentary about Gray – *And Everything Is Going Fine*, released in 2010 – he would piece the film together from existing material of Gray and without voice-over narration? No one else could speak for Spalding Gray, so why try? A documentary about someone who mercilessly self-documented may feel unnecessary. Appearing on the talk show of the now-disgraced Charlie Rose to promote *It's a Slippery Slope* – his digressive monologue about skiing – Gray was quizzed about what he doesn't confess, if anything:

> CHARLIE ROSE: What don't you put in here that you thought about? Where do you draw the line?
>
> SPALDING GRAY: Well, you know, in therapy, actually. I didn't think I could do another monologue. I pretty much almost cracked up just before this monologue.
>
> CHARLIE ROSE: Are you serious? I mean, come on?
>
> SPALDING GRAY: Yeah, was told I was manic-depressive. Was on clonopine and lithium and seeing a top psychopharmacologist here in New York City.
>
> CHARLIE ROSE: Are you serious?

SPALDING GRAY: Yeah, yeah … I don't know if that monologue gives a flavour of crack-up. Skiing really gave me a sense of balance in the middle of that crack-up.

There is something kind of aw-shucks charming about Charlie Rose's incredulity towards Gray's confession, but also something that speaks to the time in which it was made – not so long ago, of course.

—

In the popular sitcom *The Nanny*, Gray played Dr Jack Miller, Fran Drescher's character's therapist. His performance of the opposite side of the mental health industry divide is let down by the hokey nature of the show's jokes, but I do wonder what was going on in Gray's mind as he played doctor to Drescher's neurotic helper. What on earth did Gray think about playing a psych?

—

Psychoanalyst and author Darian Leader writes in *Strictly Bipolar* of his approach to writing about the lives of manic depressives: 'To explore the experience of mania, we need to listen to these accounts carefully, avoiding vague equations of noisy or elated behaviour with mania as such. Several motifs seem ubiquitous here: the sense of connectedness with other people and with the world; the spending of money, which the person usually does not have; the large appetite, be it for food, sex or words; the reinvention of oneself, the creation of a new persona as if one were someone else.'

The symptoms of manic depression, time and time again, obscure the whole view of the individual experiencing the disorder. The creation of a 'new persona' is part distraction. But this doesn't apply to everyone. Spalding Gray wasn't so much creating a new persona, in Leader's sense, but rather becoming himself. There was – as might be true in my case – a compulsive level of truth-telling, of not hiding anything, which, in itself, can be its own strategic deflection.

Gray's process of truly becoming Spalding Gray was to reduce everything down to being, practically, just him. The monologues are an internal thought process made external, and are told by a singular voice, but just on a visual level, Gray knew that things needed to be sparse in his performances to come fully into focus: there is a desk, a microphone, a glass of water, a notebook and Spalding Gray. The objects become small, unnoticeable accomplices in telling the story, of which nothing gets in the way. This reduction creates a sense of the personal, engendering an immediate and authentic connection with the audience.

—

In his landmark book *A Mood Apart: Depression, Mania, and Other Afflictions of the Self*, Dr Peter C Whybrow shows he is extremely sympathetic and in tune with the disruptions of the self for those who suffer mania. Whybrow knows that language is central to this development, and that the mimicking of language by the child leads to the adult self's eventual mastery of talk. The development of self might be a lifelong negotiation in some respects, but we collectively know that childhood and adolescence does much of the work. That might be obvious, but I mention it to emphasise that the majority of emergent manic episodes occur right at the end of this process, between the ages of twenty-one and twenty-five.

This was true for me. That this disruption and disfiguration of the self occurs at a time when those around you assume that self to be fixed in place and performing all the new adult expectations (moving out of home, securing ongoing employment, managing finances and developing adult relationships) makes the pain all the sharper.

Emily Martin writes, 'When one is diagnosed with manic-depression, one's status as a rational person is thrown into question.' You split somewhere down the middle and become two imprecise halves: one roughly rational, one largely irrational. Your life, then, becomes two possible states. Spalding Gray saw this early on, writing in his journals that there 'are at least two MES, two selves ... these two are in constant conflict'.

In a chapter of the anthology *The Self in Understanding and Treating Psychological Disorders*, titled 'The Self in Bipolar Disorder', the psychologist Nuwan D Leitan writes that 'Mania or hypomania ... may be associated with a diminished subjective experience in the world due to the body and behavior becoming separated from an individual's sense of self; correspondingly the self becomes distorted.'

I have become distorted. There are symptoms of mania that transfigure the self in dramatic ways. Delusions of grandeur can remake you as someone else entirely – mine were pretty mild. I emailed people and told them I could do their job better than they could, even though I was under-qualified, or even unqualified, for the role.

This should not have been the case: I was an extremely shy and mild-mannered child, and continued as an introverted and reserved teenager. I had my moments of extroversion – at parties, getting drunk at fourteen, or talking about whatever film came up as a topic of discussion. As I went through high school, and realised I had a kind of talent for opinion in English class – talking about books no one else in the class had read – I got a little more boisterous, enjoying argumentative and informed positions. But nothing pointed towards mania. My personality was on track, my self seemed secure. Then it wasn't. This might have been learned behaviour. At one of my earliest appointments with a psychologist – in the back of the local general practioner's office, a room that stank of chlorine and disinfectant – I sat with a woman who I did not particularly like and didn't want to trust. In desperation, I went along with whatever she said. I nodded along, bombed out of my mind in a fugue state. She made an interesting point to me in one session: 'Anxiety is contagious.' This wasn't my fault! I had caught it from someone else. Unfortunately, I told the person I thought I had caught it from, and they lost their mind. The neural network on which we all exist is pretty fragile, it turns out. I shouldn't have tested this fact.

What is definitely catching is a kind of mania for telling your own story – for becoming the kind of self-obsessed required to think that your story is even worth listening to in the first place, and to also go: I want to be an authority on this, I want to be taken seriously in the first place and for you not to give up your attention, don't give up your fix on me, or your faith in me.

—

What is it to piece together a personality during manic periods, especially given that they typically first occur just as one is coming into adulthood? The mania magnifies the best and worst of you, yes, but as you make things bigger they tend to break apart – a spall, for Spalding – and what are you left with, exactly? For me, it's a question: how do you develop a sense of self when you suffer from a disorder, which, by nature, fragments personality and disrupts the very characteristics that go towards identifying a 'self'? This question might be the very beating heart of this book. How did I form a 'self' while coming to terms with my personality being disfigured by crippling disorders? Whybrow writes that 'Depression and mania are disabilities of the mind' and this seems more true to me than just about anything else.

—

I had the desire to put on a theatrical adaptation of one of Spalding Gray's works as a revival, to explore his work in a more lived-in way. But I had no performance skills, no connections in the industry, and no idea as to how to go about it. Could I even learn a single line of dialogue? My obsession with mimicry might finally come in handy. But who would want to come and see such a work? Does Gray have any cachet any more? I did dream of wearing his combination of white sneakers, blue jeans and red flannelette shirts on stage, and sitting down at the isolated wooden desk and chair, becoming myself as many eyes were on me. I could not sell tickets, of course; not without getting the permission of his estate. Is that how theatre works? Had anyone performed Spalding Gray's work without being Spalding Gray? I looked into contacting the estate. It felt like the right thing to do, and wouldn't I need to contact them for permission for using quotes for this book anyway?

The most authentic way to get to know Spalding Gray's collected writing would be to become extremely anxious about it; to live in its anxieties by ruining your own nervous system. I called around to find a venue to put on the show. There were different options, but I really wanted the smallest, darkest room possible to hide away in, the very opposite of having people put their eyes on me.

Why would I do this though when I have my own story?

—

The story of Spalding Gray has a lovely little coda: he became a colour. I resisted writing about Gray for this book for a while simply because he did seem somewhat colourless. In many ways he presented as bland – he seemed to wear the same haircut through most of his life, prematurely grey; he had a conventionally handsome face and adopted a uniform look of jeans, sneakers and flannel shirts. He looked a bit like my dad in the 80s in these outfits. In 2001, however, the architect John Williams approached a house paint manufacturer – Sherwin Williams – with the idea of creating a paint whose colour would be taken from the colouring of his dog's coat of dullish grey fur. The dog, a Weimaraner, was named after Spalding Gray. According to the *New York Times*, in an interview with Sue Wadden, the director of colour marketing at Sherwin Williams, the colour has since become 'consistently ranked among the top 20 per cent of all [colours] sold'. The profile goes on to detail his widow Kathleen Russo's decision to paint her house 'Spalding Gray'. This fact might appear from the outside to have little to do with mania, but Gray was amazed by the connections and coincidences in the world – an ability to see these so clearly comes from mania, surely – and the fact that a dog became a colour became him became the outside of the house that homes his widow, well. That would not be lost on his hypersensitive mind, and is a testament to his character and legacy, both.

8
THE RECKONING

On a Sunday night in early October 2015, as the Grand Final of the NRL* played out on the national stage, a smaller story but a bigger fight went down. Andrew 'Joey' Johns – the former captain of the Newcastle Knights (responsible for their glorious 1997 win of the big title) – was dumped from the live coverage line-up of said Grand Final by the powers that be at Channel 9. He was removed from both a pre-game discussion panel, and the game coverage itself. It was a response to an incident that might well have been very far out of Johns' control. On the Friday night before the big game at Toowoomba Aiport, Johns was reportedly heavily intoxicated and allegedly harassed a woman sitting by herself, before setting up a makeshift camp to sleep off the booze before the flight. The woman took to her Facebook page in a small act of digital activism and lobbied Channel 9, through their *Today* show page. The woman didn't call for his sacking or removal from the NRL coverage, but she did reprimand him for his behaviour. She was calling for a change in NRL and media culture: 'I wish the Football commentators have [sic] more pride and a much higher standard of behaviour in public.'

She wasn't in the wrong. She complained to his employer, without a specific call to action. Instead, she made a call for a change in the culture of the media at large – commentators et al – and within sports reportage and for that she should be commended.

However, Andrew Johns lives with bipolar disorder and has done so since at least 2007, when he publicly came out with the diagnosis. Manic depression has yet to be brought in the disability community tent fully, but on the extreme scale it has hallucinatory and psychosis symptoms similar to schizophrenia (usually diagnosed as Bipolar 1). Bipolar 2, at the other end of the scale, is less extreme but only in symptoms. Its effects and impacts on the sufferer's life can be just as large. Both Bipolar 1 and 2 could be termed invisible illnesses and, indeed, invisible disabilities.

Back in 2007, Johns had revealed to the *Sydney Morning Herald* that he had repeatedly thought about taking his own life. Following a scandal in which he was arrested in London, Johns first considered suicide during a five-hour stint behind bars. Then, freed, he was cornered and trapped again by the media outrage that followed. In his autobiography, *The Two of Me*, he wrote:

> There were media out the front of my house. Some were ringing the doorbell on the front wall … I was on my own, pacing the house, going up and down the stairs, looking out the curtains, a prisoner in my own home with journalists and TV cameras parked on the footpath outside. That's when I became close to being suicidal. I consciously thought of taking my own life.

The woman could not see the illness that plagues Johns, despite it being on the public record. This is true of many people who encounter the effects of manic depression without knowing its root causes. The fact that the media picked up her photograph of Johns sleeping off the effects of alcohol – likely taken on her phone and almost certainly without his permission – underscores this. Plainly: if this had have been someone with a physical disability there would be no way that this photographic intrusion would be socially acceptable and so widely distributed.

The woman went on to write in a Facebook post, 'Disgusting, disgraceful and a very bad example for all to see.' She is, of course, not wrong. But Johns' behaviour, while not excusable because of his illness, is still a noted symptom of the illness. Drug and alcohol abuse are comorbid factors in manic depression. This is not always possible to see. Psychological illnesses of this kind – particularly mood disorders – are hard to explain, hard to excuse, hard to parse, just plain hardcore.

I write this because, of course, because my skin is in the game.

What I wanted to say on the night the news broke was something about what it means in practical terms for someone who grapples with mania: if I drink, I drink a lot. If I want to have sex, I want to have sex a lot. If I get angry, I get really fucking mad. If I get sad, I can't get out of bed. If I get happy, I may very well end up stealing your car and driving it across state lines.

You have to ask: is this how Johns sees himself? He has the added pressure of being in the public eye – the Facebook post and its virality proved just how public that eye can be – and the pressure of being a former sportsman, not just a role model but an 'immortal' (an NRL term for the eight greatest players of all time and invoked in the *Sydney Morning Herald*'s report on the incident). Johns proved incredibly self-aware in his autobiography; following his admissions he wrote:

> I'm not disclosing this to get any sympathy or to make
> the media feel guilty. It's not easy admitting a tough,
> big-shot footballer was on the verge of suicide because
> he'd got some bad headlines. But it's fact, part of my
> story.

In 2013, John Lehmann, editor-at-large for the *Daily Tele-graph*, wrote an op-ed under the title 'Time for troubled Andrew Johns to "man up"'. It's telling that the sub-editors put 'man up' in quotation marks. There is no 'manning up' here. The outdated gender rhetoric evoked by Lehmann is extremely unhelpful and, worse, it erases Johns' condition and sets back any subtlety in the conversation.

In any case, Johns called the woman to apologise, which must have been no easy repentance. He challenged the woman's claim that he passed out, but said she accepted his apology. The woman at Toowoomba Aiport that night was caught in a terrible intersection between sexual harassment and psychiatric disability. Unfortunately, the media are happy to turn on those who suffer from these kinds of invisible illnesses and forget, or deliberately ignore, standards of reporting on mental illness.

This isn't any one person's fault: it's the fault of a media who too easily turn to shaming as their modus operandi. Andrew Johns and the entire manic depressive community deserve better. As a close friend and ally put it in an email following the incident, 'The woman and Johns were both victims of the disorder that night'. That observation is as precise as it is incisive, because plainly this isn't a black and white issue; and it certainly isn't as simple as there being two poles to go back and forth between. Ultimately, this is only the start of a much bigger conversation in which we need to partake.

—

There is a reckoning with everything that has come before – versions of this divided and unstable self – that simply must take place at some point, because there is a 'dark backing' to every experience. In *Humboldt's Gift*, Bellow writes that 'Death is the dark backing that a mirror needs if we are to see anything.' The 'dark backing' of manic-depression – its violence, the pain it causes others, and something close to death but not quite the same thing as death – and it cannot be ignored if we are to look at any other part of it. I do not seek forgiveness, but I walk willingly towards some kind of resolve. That walk is a long, lonesome trudge through murk and, with this fucking condition being chronic, it constitutes a lifetime of walking. I will do my best not to flinch. I submit.

—

There is routine humiliation and there is a trial by fire. And there is this account. There is an admission price – a heavy toll – to the telling, and I want you to know I could have just as easily not written this chapter. We go on because we must. I could have just as easily not written the whole book, I guess, but I will pay the price, whatever it costs.

—

There is a growing self-awareness, and the responsibility and accountability that it awakens with it. I thought about this deeply while watching Andrew Johns' public humiliation unfold. The words of the late writer and editor Kat Muscat rang through my head like deafening bells:

> It is often said that people *are* their actions. Even if this can be pretty harsh, I do dig this approach to judging people (an important pastime), though it's also not cut-and-dry in its damnation. For example, if you do something shitty then apologise properly for it and don't do that shitty thing again, that's the action that defines you. Makes you a generally decent human being and whatever, which is lovely. However, what happens when our mental illness or dependency issues cause us to lose a critical level of agency? Those closest to me have had to accept many, many apologies, knowing the trigger for my objectively shitty behaviour is something that's not going to change in the foreseeable future.

Kat Muscat wrote those words for a trilogy of pieces dealing with her diagnosis with Borderline Personality Disorder for the small independent Australian literary journal *Stilts*. We lost her shortly after. Her death ripped a bright rent in the fabric of a fragile community. We have not recovered and hold onto her clear message in this piece for a structural change needing to take place within us. It calls on the media, for active witnesses, for sufferers, for medical practitioners, for carers, for the lovers, for the fighters, and for the sufferers to take part in this change.

—

The blurring of the lines is limitless. Where does the illness begin, and the behaviour end? Where does the illness begin, and character emerge? Where does the illness begin, and personality take shape? A question is a kind of reckoning, but it needs a resolve.

—

Delmore Schwartz was no good to his wife. He was violent. He apparently ran her down in a car, an incident briefly described in *Humboldt's Gift*. These are sufferings only known in private, which leak, like slick black oil, into the public sphere, spreading a toxic film over everything. They make one question everything that has come before. How do we reckon with these incursions, how do we excise them and commune with their facts?

—

I remember first watching the uploaded video of Jason Russell, screaming nude on the streets of San Diego, in a cramped office I was renting in Redfern, hired from a local literary organisation, and which I certainly could not afford. I walked in there with the intent to write, but for whatever reason, I spent most of the day on Twitter, or watching short YouTube videos. Russell's video didn't really register at the time as an overt expression of mania. But soon enough, I was watching on repeat a similar video – although this time captured by a fixed security camera – of the Australian film actor and director, Matthew Newton, in a Miami hotel lobby, assaulting a concierge in April of 2012. The raw footage was extremely disturbing, but as it had no sound, it became strangely hypnotic and, most eerily, it was somehow calming. Newton would be in the news soon enough for multiple charges of criminal activity, and his diagnosis of Bipolar Affective

Disorder would be discussed *ad nauseam* by his lawyer and the media working in a flat commentary mode. The footage of Newton provides a clear view of the darker side of mania: its swings towards physical expression and madness that has a clearer, more direct impact on others.

—

Matthew Newton, the son of the TV superstars Bert and Patti Newton,[†] came out with his bipolar diagnosis in 2012. Newton had been convicted of several instances of domestic violence towards multiple former partners. He had escaped Australia after a lot of media attention and based himself in America when the incident in the Miami hotel occurred. This was preceded by an altercation with police at a nearby bar, in which he was refused service. The details were relayed and broadcast back home as salacious media bites. To counter this, a team of lawyers were deployed to offer alternative accounts and stress Newton's diagnosis. There was a slow car crash quality to it all. Bert and Patti agreed to a misguided interview, quickly followed by Matthew giving a confusing interview on *60 Minutes*. Many people speculated he was on drugs. For the tabloid news program *A Current Affair* a dramatic voice-over claimed that Newton would tell 'the truth, the whole truth, and nothing but the truth'. He disclosed that he was taken to a psychiatric ward and escaped, before a thundering sound effect was dropped over the top of his confession.

In the resulting interview with the tabloid TV program, Newton admitted to throwing himself against walls. In a write-up based on the interview, Newton was reported as having said 'he had thrown himself at floors and walls as he went through therapy as well as dislocating his jaw and putting a fist through a window, doing damage that required micro surgery'. Things have to be very bad indeed to break your own jaw.

—

In an even-handed opinion piece written for the *Newcastle Herald*, the journalist and Newcastle Writers Festival director Rosemarie Milsom reflected on Newton's public trial and the confusion and furore surrounding his diagnosis:

> Those with a mental illness have voiced concern that Newton's violent behaviour boosts misunderstanding about bipolar disorder, which is defined as a set of mood swing conditions, the most severe form of which used to be called 'manic depression'. It is a debilitating illness, but it can be managed – with a high standard of psychiatric care, a cocktail of medication, and the support of family and friends. Most importantly, the person with the disorder needs to have insight into their condition. This all sounds marvellous in theory, but if you have ever observed a loved-one struggle with bipolar disorder it quickly becomes clear that the winning formula for maintaining well-being can be frustratingly elusive, even impossible. Add addiction to the equation – as in Newton's case – and there is another level of complexity.

Complexity is the right word. Domestic violence cannot and should not be excused in any way, but discussing Newton is important, as he brought the disorder into the mainstream spot-light, and though the debates around his multiple confessions

were ugly, they were, ultimately, telling. In his televised interview, Newton, looking desperate, spoke to the camera: 'It's like
you want to rip your brain out of your head, put it under a tap,
wash it clean, and then put it back in the skull.'‡

I cannot think of a better description for all of this.

—

This is not to play the part of the apologist – a role that too
easily leads one to becoming a queasy moralist and absolutist.
Though it is important to state clearly: self-harm is real.
Mostly when we say self-harm, we think of cutting, which
leaves visible marks. My wounds were invisible, and not lasting. I would punch myself repeatedly on the side of the head
in moments when I couldn't contain the multitudes of my
selves.

—

Watching the Australian film *Lion*, tears flooded down my
face. The film is a sob-fest, yes, but I was crying for a number
of reasons. Coming home from the film, I wrote this social
media post on my phone:

> TW: Self harm.
> So, *Lion* is a masterpiece. Who knew? My best mate
> Bina Bhattacharya has a much stronger personal
> connection to it, of course, as I imagine many people
> who have come from Indian families [have], as well as
> those from diverse parts of Asia. But I found a personal
> connection in there too, in its subtle depiction of mental
> ill health, which it gets scarily spot on. Both in Nicole
> Kidman's incredible portrayal of an all-too-familiar

dead-eyed depression, and more importantly, the manic self-harm of the main character's brother, portrayed incredibly (if only briefly) by Divian Ladwa in his adult iteration. Spoiler alert but two unrelated children are adopted by Kidman's character, and the second adopted brother clearly struggles with some variation of either Bipolar Affective Disorder or Borderline Personality Disorder, with PTSD almost certainly mixed in. Unfortunately, one common symptom of these disorders is self-harm; I have experienced this in a personal manner, in a way that is very similar to how it is depicted in the film – a repetitive violent hitting of one's own head, with either an object or your own fists. In fact, I experienced it yesterday, an unfortunate flare-up due to environmental stress and ongoing professional conflict. Consider it like a form of physical Tourette's syndrome, but it's basically uncontrollable for me without some form of mood-stabilising medication. It's not something I choose to do, to put it basically. Anyway, as I was sitting in the cinema bawling my eyes out, a couple of women behind me snickered at this depiction … It took everything in my power to not go full mentally ill mutant and turn around and scream at them, but it just goes to show – and I only relate the story here for this reason – that there remains an incredible amount of stigma towards such conditions, and a huge gap in people's understandings. Radical, transparent honesty/vulnerability and all that: I'm okay but the last couple of months have been tough. I've basically sprained my foot kicking a wall. But life's like that. Anyway, go see *Lion*, give all your good movie money to it, because it's breaking down multiple barriers in the space of a couple of hours, both for people from CALD backgrounds and those who suffer from mental ill health! Two for the price of one! Bring a couple of boxes of tissues though, wooooooooooooooooooowee it's a bawl-your-eyes-out fest.

The film's screenwriter, Australian poet and novelist Luke Davies, responded to this after being tagged in the post by a mutual friend. He kindly said he would pass on my words to the rest of the cast and crew. I sighed a breath of relief – this is the reckoning doing its work.

—

There is the cold acknowledgment that some things you will never get right, particularly in the imprecise art of writing, or its fumbling ugly attempts. There is messy reality, and there are times when it only ever seems to come that way.

—

There is a self-destructive drive and its ownership. The literature of this self-destructiveness is too vast to even attempt to view as a whole. There's no point shuffling up to an active volcano and peering in over the edge. And besides it is too strewn with the same lit dude bro names who appear over and over again. It is, however, worth singling out Frederick Exley's *A Fan's Notes*. Published in 1968, the novel is broadcast as a 'fictional memoir', taking in Exley's years of alcoholism and time spent in mental institutions. It is the reckoning with the self of the kind I had long been searching for. During an admission to an emergency ward due to a seizure, Exley reflects:

> Unlike some men, I had never drunk for boldness or
> charm or wit; I had used alcohol for precisely what
> it was, a depressant to check the mental exhilaration
> produced by extended sobriety.

The tension in *A Fan's Notes* is that the technical quality of the writing does not quite match the state of the autobiographical figure – often drunk, flailing about. Lucidity is sometimes given most to those for whom it can be out of reach on bad days. You have to ask: did he write this drunk? There's a genuine listlessness to the book for most of its length – the listlessness is the thing itself, its artistry is in making a lack of conviction into an object driven by conviction (the novel) – so, a few beers in would create that rambling think-speak that takes up most of its rhetorical forward movement. Did I write drunk? No, I could not manage it.

In the hospital, the doctor standing over me, his face stern and unmoving, intimidation his bedside manner of choice, asked: 'How much did you drink tonight?' I forgot that I had had anything to drink at all, so caught up in the sweep of mania. 'Ten beers, maybe more, at a guess.' There had also been the pack of cigarettes, moved through like a force: all smoked in the single sitting, ushering through thought as talk at a fast rate. Was it just the alcohol, after all that, that had spun things askew? At that count, very likely. Maybe I've just been drunk and lilting the whole time.

The American academic Peter Bailey had his thoughts on *A Fan's Notes* quoted in David Shields' *Reality Hunger*, having noted that 'Frederick seems, throughout the course of the narrative, to be writing – or trying to write – the very book we're reading. Which accounts for the greater technical and structural complexity of *A Fan's Notes* and also explains why a book so carefully created and meticulously ironised was so often criticised for being autobiographically self-indulgent.' Exley's categorisation of the book as a 'fictional memoir' creates the right feeling for this tension, but the designation points not only to the book itself, but the life sitting a little out of sight, right behind it.

Drug and alcohol abuse is common amongst manic-depressives. We have ended up calling it 'self-medicating'. Alcoholism runs through my family. An uncle shaved his head and took a whipper-snipper into the grounds of Wollongong University with the hopes of terrorising his father, a mathematics professor. Anatole Broyard writes that Malcolm Lowry 'uses the delirium of illness in *Under the Volcano*, where alcohol is the consul's disease ... "a fever of matter", like a slip or glitch in our composition ...'

There is that violence again, and how to survive it. In *Strictly Bipolar* – which Hilary Mantel classified as 'a contribution to a debate' but one that 'could also change lives' – Darian Leader writes: 'Any situation that involves violence and hate may stir up this motif of responsibility, and hence the importance of protecting the Other from harm. As a patient put it, "It's not so much the aggression as the fact that people will think it's my aggression".'

So there is the deep horror at being seen as violent, as if an ideal of pacifism has to be maintained at all costs.

In his book, *Depression and How to Survive It*, co-authored with noted manic depressive Spike Milligan, the Irish TV psychiatrist Anthony Clare took a discomforting magnifying lens to Milligan's life. Milligan suffered an enormous number of breakdowns during his lifetime, and the book is largely concerned with the creative connections contained within his illness. However, Clare crafts a conflicting portrait of the well-loved Milligan, and the man he meets in a depressive state – a cantankerous, biting subject, who demonstrates as much misanthropy as one good doctor can stomach. Milligan spouts racist drivel and nasty nonsense and rails against overpopulation (despite having a good number of children himself). Clare is calm throughout his transcribed sessions, and reflects towards the middle of the book on Milligan's potential for violent outbursts and verbal lashings. Clare knows, as many mental health professionals do, that manic-depressives are not, on the whole, violent. Much stigma of mental ill health arises from such misconceptions. Clare admits that 'manic individuals can behave in a reckless and disinhibited way and, if crossed, can be irritable, abusive and even violent'. But he writes forcefully about the counterpoint to this view:

> One of the difficulties that bedevils psychiatric illness
> is its association in the public mind with violence.
> People fear the emotional disturbance because they
> fear its unpredictability, its explosiveness. In fact, the
> overwhelming majority of psychologically stressed
> individuals are not violent and are probably more in

danger of their own lives at the hands of the so-called normal than the normal are at the hands of them.

The urtext of these manic confessions was a VHS copy of a Spike Milligan documentary about depression in my local library. I spied it on the shelves as a child and never borrowed it, but I looked at the cover a lot. The book came later. I was sceptical about *Depression and How to Survive It* at first, but on a recent close reading, found its unique structure – Clare interviews Milligan in great depth and detail about his psychiatric history – definitively useful. To subject yourself to public scrutiny – bringing into question your likeability and difficultness – isn't necessarily a brave thing to do, but it is extremely beneficial to the world at large. Milligan's body of work counters the horrors of the twentieth century, bringing humour to the atrocities of the Second World War. So, why not look into the horrors of your very being?

For me, there was a feeling of proximity and familiarity with Milligan: he looked like my uncles and cousins, and there had always been a tongue-in-cheek extroverted energy to members of my family. Even my grandmother looked like him. She housed several of his books in her limited library. There was a literal proximity too: his parents had, famously, moved to Woy Woy,** on the same stretch of the Central Coast between Sydney and Newcastle where I had grown up, and he visited them often. In my mind, he visited them during depressive episodes, where, in a sleepy riverside town, he could escape everyone. I thought a lot about the mangroves in the mud of Woy Woy, their roots submerged in grey, murky mush. Looking out on that scene must have legitimised many low moods – sometimes in the midst of depression you seek out the monochromatic in everything, to reflect your own colourlessness.

One of my first appointments with a psychologist took place in Woy Woy. I took comfort in the fact that Spike Milligan, that most famous of manic depressives, had come to Woy Woy to rest up and live down his mania during his extreme mood swings and managed not to kill himself while there. Watching videos of Milligan on YouTube were my only source of pleasure in those grim weeks. His energy and the speed at which he moved gave me hope, as I paced the house in a turgid state of mind. They had named a local bridge after Milligan, but it was the straightest, most boring bridge ever invented, capturing none of Milligan's erratic personality. It made me depressed just walking over it, but I could go deeper by looking to the other side of the township, where the water was a murky shitty brown and the mangroves drooped into the mud.

Milligan had darkly quipped that Woy Woy was the biggest above-ground cemetery in Australia, having a dig at the elderly population, but he later revised and simplified those dark jibes to the following: 'Woy Woy is a good place to commit suicide'. I hadn't consulted any of the biographies at that point and did not know the real reasons for Milligan's depression while in Woy Woy.

—

There is self-doubt, and self-abnegation. Is there any other illness that has as a symptom, 'Makes you into a raging arse-hole'? Someone close to me, years after having helped me through a manic episode, confessed that, in private, she had referred to it as 'the Arsehole Disease'.

—

Kristin Ohlson, a science writer, observes in a moving, short memoir about her friend, titled *Unravelling Man*: 'He became hypomanic, although I didn't use such an alarming clinical term to describe it. *Annoying* is the word I used.'

—

I have been deeply, deeply annoying to others, and to myself.

—

There is the clean-up after an episode. It is left largely to the sufferer and their closest relations – those who can't get away from the wreckage. A reckoning with this self, and what one has done, must take place to get things back in order, and it's very hard not to fall into a depression when surveying the damage. Relationships are destroyed. The fragility of friendships can feel like thin glass, and you are a rattling wind against the windows. The manic depressive knows more about the impact of conflict – things said, and unsaid – than anyone else.

—

I am not a good person. This would not be such a painful admission if moral complexity were more prized in the mainstream culture, a vision that seems out of reach in a country that eulogises endlessly and at length without really thinking what it is that is truly dead.

—

There are, unfortunately, other people. They have to be contended with.

—

People get angry. People get upset with other people. But there is inherent risk in that tipping over, and of it, in fact, triggering a manic episode. So you mute yourself, or when you are angry you hide yourself away.

—

I recall reading on my way home from work – my first stable job since diagnosis – about the Sydney magistrate, Brian Vincent Maloney,[††] who was battling to keep his job on the bench, after a Judicial Commission of NSW report had found that he had acted 'well below the standard of a judicial officer'. The report was tabled to the NSW Parliament following four complaints against Maloney. According to the reporting in the *Sydney Morning Herald* article, Maloney 'was found to have ridiculed and bullied an unrepresented litigant and urged a pregnant psychiatric registrar to stand up and show how pregnant she was'.

In judgment of the case, 'His Honour found that the evidence of Dr Nielssen, with which the other two doctors agreed, was that on balance, Magistrate Maloney would be the subject of at least one (1) further hypomanic episode during his working career as a magistrate. If not detected and treated immediately, this could lead to behaviour that was unjudicial.'

Maloney was ordered to make his case to the upper house of the NSW Parliament, and standing in front of its members, spoke of his diagnosis. For him it was 'An illness I did not choose to have, but one I acquired. I unconditionally accept the diagnosis and take up the challenge to conquer it.'

Brian Vincent Maloney survived being put up for the vote to remove him from the bench (MPs voted, finding that his bipolar disorder had not impaired his judgment, and were satisfied that he was sufficiently medicated), but he died just two years after this incident, and just six months after receiving a life-saving heart transplant. His body took in the new heart initially, after a five-hour operation and with no signs of rejecting the organ, but he succumbed to an infection. This was the dark backing of his mirror.

—

I deeply sympathised with Maloney's position at the time. Manic depression means I too have been overly susceptible to professional conflict. For three years I worked as CEO and artistic director of a writers' festival in Melbourne. That city's passion for the arts leads it to many excesses – the festival, when I took it over, ran for eleven days on a skeleton staff. Running an underresourced festival of that length was not good for my illness. The job and its punishing schedule created havoc with my calendar year – and, in fact, in many ways it mimicked those old bipolar swings (months of excitement in pre-planning, the manic energy of the festival itself, and then the crashing lows after it ends, when everyone packs up and goes home and forgets to thank you for your work). The chair of the board talked about 'post-festival blues'.

—

It is a lot to ask of someone to be able to distinguish between the illness and its effects, and the person beneath. Forgiveness can be hard to come by. It is a sign of great intelligence and

195

kindness when people can. Others get clouded by their own emotional past, and if you're asking forgiveness you should probably learn to forgive yourself.

Witness is important, and I craved it. On a night before I was hospitalised, I screamed and hit the carpet beneath my fists: 'I want them to see what they've done.' I repeated this many times. I wasn't so paranoid. I really did want 'them' to see what they had done. In my mind, the episode needed witness to become real.

—

There is anxiety: as I came towards the end of writing this essay, I had a horrible anxiety dream in which I was accused of using 'bipolar' as an excuse for bad behaviour – for doing the evils that can come from being a white man in a position of power. I felt aghast through this dream – accused by a writer who I've never met, but followed on social media – and I woke up in a sweat. Walking off the fear, I thought, this could come true once this book is published. It is possible. I will not lie: there is a deep temptation to weaponise the diagnosis in this way. It is a reality. I live with this, like many others diagnosed with severe mood disorders, and will continue to do so until the day I die. Writing this provides no real relief, but opens an uncomfortable enquiry that will go on for some time to come. I can only say, I dare to look into the darkness, and I might not be right about what I see there.

—

So, there is a reckoning, and it is no one person's responsibility and no one person's liability and no one person's accountability. It does not wholly lie with those who have been diagnosed as manic depressive, and demonstrated bad behaviour. It lies also with those on the other side of the mirror – those who encounter us when we are at our most out of control and in need of saving.

* The NRL is the National Rugby League, a game primarily popular in New South Wales and Queensland, and not to be confused with the Australian Football League.

† Bert Newton (born 1938) is a famous Australian television personality who was immensely popular from the 1950s until the 1990s. He married his co-worker Patti in 1974 and the couple became media darlings.

‡ In 2018, Matthew Newton was removed as director of a green-lit film project set to star Jessica Chastain, after the American press uncovered Newton's past instances of domestic violence in Australia. It is important to stress that people who suffer from mental illnesses are statistically more likely to be the victims of violence than the perpetrators – and, while studies are inconclusive in regards to links between bipolar and aggressive behaviour, there is evidence of links between the two, particularly during the manic or mixed-state phases. While bipolarity and psychosis can be an obvious root cause for extremes of anti-social behaviour, it is important not to ignore the severe impacts that these behaviours have on others and, speaking only for myself, risk assessment when entering into new work arrangements can certainly be warranted if fairly and indiscriminately executed.

** Woy Woy is a small coastal town on the southern end of the Central Coast region in New South Wales.

†† Brian Vincent Maloney (1952–2013) was a Sydney-based judge.

9
CARRIE F
[OCTOBER 21, 1956–DECEMBER 27, 2016]

[2017]
Dear Carrie, this one is for you.

[2018]
Well, it's *about* you, which I'm not sure is quite the same thing as being *for* you, but it is for you, really it is.

[2015]
'I think in my mouth, so I don't lie.'

[1977]
Here we go: Carrie Fisher came into being twice. The first was as an actress who landed, at the age of nineteen, the kind of role that has less to do with acting than with a perpetual non-stop proliferation of an image, an incessant iconography that removes selfhood and deifies until you're made sick. (Is it obvious that I'm talking about Princess Leia from those *Star Wars* films?) So, you are living in the shadow of some images of you playing dress-ups at age nineteen. Your real life is hedonism afforded by those images and pushed on you by the attention too. There was a doll-like quality to these performances – made literal by her likeness being used to create plastic toys to

sell to children, a joke she would make again and again in later life, railing against George Lucas and the commercial powers that be. In a 2005 riotous roast of Lucas, as part of an AFI Life Achievement ceremony, Fisher opened with the lines 'Hi, I'm Mrs Han Solo and I'm an alcoholic. I'm an alcoholic because George Lucas ruined my life.' She didn't soften from there. This was a consistent characteristic of her public life. There was a toughness and shrewdness to her Princess Leia, qualities she brought to the role and lived out too as she rebelled against commercial spotlighting, subverting it across her career.

[1956]
She was famous from the start – her mother was movie star Debbie Reynolds and her father was the singer Eddie Fisher – and then, a second wave of fame hit, built on the unexpected success of *Star Wars*, a film that would change the way we consume cinema. She was defined through the lens. And she used it to her advantage – after coming out as a manic depressive and detailing her drug addiction, she found the outlets usually afforded to 'stars' as a place to humanise not only herself but the struggles of others. Her advocacy was found in late-night television appearances. And some breakfast morning chatter. And the occasional award show or valourising lifetime achievement program.

[1977]
Is this all illusion?

[1987]
The second emergence coincided with the publication of *Postcards from the Edge*. Released in her thirty-first year, the

book is a tell-all, semi-autobiographical novel, about an actress named Suzanne Vale. The book is restless in form – skipping between letters, diary entries and dialogue. Classic third-person omniscient narration doesn't make its entrance until more than a third of the way through.

Let us also praise what was at risk – a career, the formulation of an identity based on work and a creative image. To turn to writing when she was so well known for another artform in another category entirely is no small feat.

She was already known as a great talker and a great wit. Is it any wonder, then, that the best stretch of the book is a long dialogue between Suzanne and an unnamed producer that unfolds like a more pop, sex-obsessed LA version of *My Dinner with Andre*? The novels don't quite cohere, but they are filled with enthusiasms and powerful digressions and insight. I might not be overly impressed with their literary qualities at all times, but the production and what they uncover gives me strength. These are not perfect fictions, but, somehow, they equate to a perfect life.

[1990]

The filmed adaptation of *Postcards from the Edge*, released in 1990, the turn of a new decade, quickly followed the book. Directed by Mike Nichols from a screenplay by Fisher, the movie is concerned with deceptions that are quickly uncovered. This trick is played out several times. The film opens on a film within the film; Meryl Streep plays Suzanne Vale, a veiled version of Carrie Fisher, playing another character in a film.

The opening scene is a delicious double fold: Streep walks through the streets of an unnamed South American country, and we think that the scene playing out is real – if a little hokey – before she flubs a line and the director, played by Gene Hackman, comes out of hiding. She takes the fake moustache off an actor playing the cop who just hit her and places it above her lip, mugging for the camera. More fiction meets reality unfolds: one of the crew members in the scene can be seen wearing a t-shirt with 'EVIL ANGELS' emblazoned on the back, referring to the film starring Streep playing Lindy Chamberlain (the film was released as *A Cry in the Dark* outside of Australia and New Zealand).

Suzanne retreats to her trailer as the scene is reset for a second attempt, and the sound guys pick up the sound of her snorting a line of coke. Hackman's director clues in and berates Suzanne. He scornfully gets in her face: 'You fuck up my movie, I'll kill you. I'll kill you before you kill yourself, and I'll do a better job because you're so out of it you'll probably botch it up.'

In the film Suzanne briefly dates a cad played by Dennis Quaid, who hooks up with Vale, and after she overdoses in his bed, drops her off at Emergency before taking off in his car. Later, Vale/Streep/Fisher gets her revenge by threatening him with a gun, which fires blanks. The cinematic trickery continues. They flirt in front of a plain house which later pulls away to be revealed as a film set. Reality is pulled away like a rug beneath our feet.

It probably wasn't all that strange for Fisher to see her life doubled on film. Her life had celluloid woven throughout – it must have been part of the everyday, waking textures. Still, seeing Meryl Streep playing some version of yourself *would* be strange. Whose memories are these?

Richard Dreyfuss, fellow manic depressive, plays the doctor who pumps Suzanne's stomach. Keep it in the family, it would seem.

[2016]
When Carrie Fisher died, a sense of immense shock ran through me. A close friend texted, 'So sorry, sweetie.' I didn't know what he was referring to until I checked the news. I had a stark realisation (one seen only through clouding tears): that Carrie Fisher was my mental health icon, for at least a decade, if not longer. I am fast coming up to a decade of living with a diagnosis of manic depression, something I don't really think about any more – although here we are – because I'm so well medicated and supported that I sort of stink of sane right now.

[1968]
Patty Duke, in the middle of an extended period of mania, found herself appearing on *The Dick Cavett Show* – her manager continued to book her for such shows, not knowing of her manic condition – and in a long rambling conversation she told the host that she was going to 'build an ark in the desert between Barstow and Bakersfield'. John Berryman's alter-ego Alan Severance, in the opening of his semi-autobiographical novel *Recovery*, lists himself as a 'twice-invited guest on the [sic] *Dick Cavett Show* (stoned once, and a riot)'. Dick Cavett himself would later go public about suffering from manic depression in 1997 when he was sued for backing out of a radio talk show and cited the disorder as his reason. Cavett, then, is another exemplar of the 'normal seeming' manic depression – his role as mediator on his syndicated talk show, as even-handed a host as you're ever likely

to see, plays its part in this view of him (anyone would look sane sitting next to, and attempting to interpret, the likes of Marlon Brando, Bette Davis, Muhammad Ali and Groucho Marx – especially if you know that Norman Mailer has just head-butted Gore Vidal backstage before carrying on their bickering in front of the cameras).

[2015]
On exiting Central Park, I asked my wife if she thought we would see any more celebrities on the trip, only to have Woody Allen appear in front of us. He was walking with Dick Cavett, and it will remain a lifelong regret that I didn't approach Cavett and ask for his signature, with my back turned to Allen.

[1962]
Duke was best known at the time for being the youngest winner of an Academy Award, given for playing Helen Keller in *The Miracle Worker*, and as a teen idol – roughly akin to Miley Cyrus's Hannah Montana stint – in her years on *The Patty Duke Show*.

[1990]
In the 1990 TV movie adaptation of Duke's memoir *Call Me Anna*, Duke agreed to play herself on screen. Two actors – Ari Meyers and Jenny Robertson – played younger versions of Duke before Duke takes over. In an interview with Oprah at the time of the film's release, Duke observed that 'something about telling somebody, or somebody reading, [about] it, is a whole generation away from demonstrating it'. Indeed, it is one thing to write a memoir or perform a monologue,

it's quite another to inhabit yourself as an actor and re-enact scenes from your own life, particularly moments that are extreme reflections of your character. Duke says that the decision to play herself lent the project a sense of 'credibility' and she's not wrong. The film has the cheesy feel of made-for-TV movies – it counts as an early screen credit for Matthew Perry ahead of being cast in the interminable *Friends* – but there's something about Duke's commitment to recreating her manic episodes that pushes it over the border into art. The movie opens at a high pitch of emotion – Duke waking her husband up, screaming and smashing a lamp. A kind of involuntary violence is evoked again later, when Duke lashes out against Christmas dinner, smashing her many meals to pieces.

[2008]
How do you play yourself? The novel became a film, and Meryl Streep plays you. The memoir becomes a stage show and you play yourself. All these selves come together eventually.

[2018]
Why is time so important to this essay – to the point it needs time markers – to me in this moment, late in writing the book? I need to measure the timeline, the beats of a life, and how and when we intersect. Psychologists make you keep mood diaries – tracing the ups and downs, day by day, to get a sense of the swings – and the diagnostic categories are all largely attempts to narrativise time. Life is also just fast – it possesses its own forms of mania – and I need to slow it down for a second.

[2008]

Carrie published the first of three book-length memoirs – the fictional curtain, or Vale, is dropped – with *Wishful Drinking* in 2008, the same year in which I was first diagnosed as a manic depressive. I didn't read the book at the time, but I was aware of an incoming stage version of the show to be performed in Sydney. I didn't go, to my permanent regret.

[2006]

In 2006, Fisher appeared in Stephen Fry's BBC documentary *The Secret Life of the Manic-Depressive* as one of the first guests he interviewed in a long line-up (Richard Dreyfuss features towards the end). This was, for me, the introduction to Fisher's history with the illness and her brand of extreme frankness when discussing her condition. I watched the documentary on YouTube, where it had been uploaded in cut-up parts. I identified so strongly with the documentary that I had forgotten I had seen it before being diagnosed. Once again with feeling: what's weird in retrospect is how I seem to have willed some of these circumstances into being; how much I seemed to know before I knew anything at all.

[2016]

When she died, time was already out of sync. The southern hemisphere summer heat was in its oppressive stage, and in my friendship group things were heating up. Indeed, part of the shock of Fisher's death was realising we had lost such a strong advocate, a voice who enunciated, with great strength and clarity, the particular costs of living with the disorder. It was easy to forget that she had been doing so for a very long time. In losing a leading light, we found, through shared mourning, the community around us. So, yes, I had my own personal rituals (screaming in the ocean on hearing of her heart attack), but then a good friend – a fellow writer and broadcaster – sent me a message on the day of her death, asking for a one-on-one beer at the quietest pub we could find, to share our feelings of loss and reflect on our own stories once more. We talked about setting up a possible cultural resource for those newly diagnosed with the disorder, a hint towards further public campaigning (indeed, Fisher herself had a similar set of resources on her website already). We hugged it out.

[2017]

I was left devastated by her death because for many of us living with the disorder she was providing a pretty terrific mud map on how to get through life with it, and, most importantly, to age with it. I mourn that she won't show us how to live through her sixties and seventies and, hypothetically, further on, but, back to reality, she has also tragically proved that we have a statistically higher risk of dying younger and not just from the complications caused by suicidal ideation.

[2008]

Wishful Drinking closes out with an earnest Author's Note: 'One of the things that baffles me (and there are quite a few) is how there can be so much lingering stigma with regards to mental illness, specifically bipolar disorder. In my opinion, living with manic depression takes a tremendous amount of balls ... At times, being bipolar can be an all-consuming challenge, requiring a lot of stamina, and a lot more courage, so if you're living with this illness and functioning at all, it's something to be proud of, not ashamed of.' Amen to that.

[2017]
She is back in the news, relevant in the post-Weinstein revelations, for having once sent a cow tongue to a producer who had sexually harassed a friend of hers; along with it a note, if you harass my friend again, or any woman, 'the next delivery will be something of yours in a much smaller box'.

[1990/1994]
Debbie Reynolds went on TV to say that the film was not about them in an interview with Larry King, wanting to correct the public record. Carrie herself offered this on an interview program with Ruby Wax: 'As soon as I've written this book, it's no longer true of me. So it always makes me laugh when people say, "Are they autobiographical?" Not any more. But they were at the time. If I'm able to say it and name it, it's no longer so, precisely.'

[ongoing]
If mania is marked by a naked narcissism and self-delusions, then when that has fallen away, it can often give way to honest self-reflection, partly in order to correct what has come before it. That can perilously tip into the obsessive self-hatred of a depressive episode, but if it does not, it can be something of a gift; to live between two extremes is to have an insight into your own character that others may never have access to. Is this where the writing comes from? Is this how Carrie Fisher could sit down and write a novel, and then a film, and then another novel and another?

Late-night television appearances are a pure form of storytelling. There is some rehearsal involved – a producer will typically seek out stories worth telling ahead of time, teasing out their rhythms and briefing the host in how to best coax them out. The same stories are told for new audiences. It is essential that there are such repeat admissions. The format is populist.

There were many appearances on British television – she frequently visited the UK, where she had studied acting as a teenager – which, despite the cultural clichés of being a reserved, stiff-upper-lip country, have programs that are far more raucous in tone than their American counterparts. The back and forth is more boisterous, capitalising on quick-wittedness.

[2016]
When she dies, I go out of my way to create a GIF from a scene in *Drop Dead Fred,* where, playing along, Fisher grabs the titular imaginary friend and wrings him by the neck – except she doesn't. He is standing away from her, and she is strangling air. That empty space could come to mean anything, and in the moment of trying to put together the images, I suppose I was hoping it would represent my silent wrestling with this star's death, while representing her own reckoning with invisible struggles.

[ongoing]
The continuing online trade of her iconography is now largely made up of photographs in which she has extended her middle finger. Her humour – how it grew out of suffering – is vital to her memory, to mine. I wish for such a loving embrace, and then to refute it with a flip of the bird. Fuck you. I love you, but, really, fuck you.

[1977 – onwards]
It was in the way that she sat on these talk shows, jumping up onto the kind of armchairs normally on offer, and tucking her feet beneath her, or sitting cross-legged. Why do I find the smallest acts the most radical? It was never really a defiance, of course, it was simply to say: I feel at home, here. And here, in the talk show sense, is your self, as that is what is ultimately on offer – not the book, or film, or record, for sale. Late-night TV self is self-constructed from anecdotes. And so, the sitting position is to say: I feel at home as myself.

There are many filmed interviews you can find in which she is on a bed with the interviewer, or subject. This speaks of comfort, but also a kind of restlessness that was such a large part of her character. In bed with the comedian Ruby Wax, feet curled up, they talk about her book *Delusions of Grandma*.

Later, she would be joined by her dog, a French bulldog named Gary, who accompanied her everywhere. Gary had the same relaxed approach to talk shows, sitting unamused throughout gabfests with his owner. The dog doesn't talk but says more than most. Gary essentially became a care animal. A friend recently applied for a permit for such status for her dog, to sit next to her in cafés while she writes. I yearn for such a relationship.

[circa 2008]
I have watched so many of her talk show appearances now that the stories have started to blur into one another, and some are, indeed, repeated over the years. One line appears again and again: 'If my life wasn't funny, it would just be true, and that's unacceptable.'

[1977 – 2016]

There was the ongoing partnership with Craig Ferguson – a late-night TV host of Scottish background – who was also a recovering alcoholic, and made frequent reference to this in public, on his show. So, that was a shared affinity for honesty. Someone understood this connection and edited together just her entrances to his program, over many years and appearances: the same embrace, a knowingness, repeated over time. There's the generosity of camaraderie right there – a shared sense of humour, but also an understanding, together, of the progress away from self-destructiveness.

[2017]

There are snatches of rare home video featured in the HBO documentary film *Bright Lights: Starring Carrie Fisher and Debbie Reynolds* (the film was screened very shortly following the deaths of both mother and daughter, the schedule moved forward to capitalise on public interest, and to provide people with a chance to reflect with the film). Carrie is walking on the Great Wall of China in 1988. She looks into the camera (it is not made clear who is holding it, but the intimacy is very strong): 'It's Christmas here on the Wall and we're headed for the top.' Carrie is carrying a pink boom box playing old show-tune versions of Christmas carols. 'Come on everybody', she calls out, before dancing with strangers, seemingly without their consent, clutching at them and making them ultra-awkward.

[2006]

It is interesting that she was cast as a wise, counselling friend in both *When Harry Met Sally* and *Drop Dead Fred*. She played a family therapist in *Austin Powers: International Man of Mystery*, counselling Dr Evil and his son. She seemed to actually take up this role in real life – I'm thinking here of her counselling the musician, actor and artist Courtney Love in the TV documentary *The Return of Courtney Love*, screened on More4 in Britain. Love visits Carrie Fisher in her eclectic Los Angeles home (which would feature in *The Secret Life of the Manic-Depressive* and *Bright Lights*). The narrator of the documentary counts Fisher as one of Love's 'greatest mentors' and notes that together they scan *Country Life* magazine, with Love looking at houses for sale in Hampshire. Love is concerned about the intrusive British tabloid paparazzi. Fisher counsels her to 'act a tabloid-free life'.

[1980s]
'We're having a ball. Well, soon that methamphetamine released itself and the brain slid and there was some trapped methamphetamine from my father ...'
    'Listen to the music. It's melting ... from the heat.'
    Later, Fisher is shown lying in a bed, curled up sick with a cold, holding a pillow, clearly exhausted but wanting to confess: 'I have two moods. Roy is rollicking Roy. A wild ride of a mood. Pam is sediment Pam who stands on the shore and sobs. One mood is the meal, the next mood the cheque. Where am I in all this? I have no idea, cause I feel like it's a little mood relay and I'm Pam now, see if Roy got this cold he wouldn't let him stop it, cause Roy is bigger than all of it, but I just fit snugly into the mood pocket that is Pam, I don't have any choice, I don't dictate the ride.'

[2000]

Creative responses to mania tend to get an easier ethical pass than attempts at documentary commentary. In an interview with the BBC program *HARDtalk with tim SEBASTIAN* (the bizarre capitalisations are theirs) for instance, Fisher is introduced, condescendingly, thus:

> In the words of my guest she had the classic Hollywood upbringing, in a beautiful but broken home. There followed a star role in *Star Wars*, and the obligatory going off the rails with drugs and divorce. Now she says she's a single parent, with a dysfunctional family all of her own. How is she now?

Carrie, moments later, after sitting through the cordial introductory remarks, calls Sebastian out. 'The obligatory going off the rails, did you say? I like that that's obligatory now. Yes, I've done that a couple of times, but I've done non-obligatory things as well.' He follows up with a dumb question about Fisher starring as Princess Leia and Fisher plays along, having picked him up on his insensitive phrasing. I and many others have, many times, called out journalists to get training in how to write about mental ill health and to avoid sensationalising language.

[2011]

A video advertisement of Carrie Fisher talking about her weight produced for Jenny Craig doesn't disclose that some of the medications have weight gain as a side effect. This is a reality for those trying to correct the condition. The current medication I am on changes the way the body stores fat.

I don't mind being slightly overweight, but it does seem to sit in a kind of cruel opposition to mania: all that fast running, shedding weight, in your mind at least. When I look in the mirror with my shirt off, I am reminded of my mind.

[2013]

Carrie's breakdown on a cruise ship – which was filmed – resonates significantly with me because a cruise ship seems like the perfect setting in which to have a manic episode. Watching video tours of cruise ships confirms this thinking: bright colours, electric screens, easy access to alcohol, eerie entertainment, and large chaotic crowds of over-eager, overly excited people. Then, of course, there's the ocean, flat and still, which at any given opportunity you could throw yourself into to cancel out all the noise. The knowledge of it being there, with some famous overboard suicides in your mind, would be enough to drive anyone to the edge. I have banned myself from cruise liners for other reasons: my grandfather died of a heart attack on one, and was buried at sea. Years later, a great uncle died on a cruise too, though by this time they had installed morgues on most ships, and he was put on ice. Male members of my family seem destined for doom by accepting this mode of leisure.

During my first ever mania – baby's first manic episode – I got addicted to playing bingo with the blue-rinse set at the local RSL, walking in with my big blue stamp pen to mark off the numbers.

[circa 2011]

Writing about mental ill health is good business, and staggeringly popular with readers. A friend, Elmo Keep, wrote an article for the Australian literary magazine *Meanjin* – 'Summer and Antipsychotics in the City' – about tripping into a bout of short-lived psychosis after being unable to sleep through a heat wave. It was the most popular essay published on that magazine's website for that year, by quite a margin.

[2004]
From a breakfast television interview on British TV: 'Too much of a good thing. There's another weird word for it, dysphoria – it's like euphoria gone terribly wrong. For me it's like mania ... like in manic depression. Mania is fantastic, right up until it isn't.'

[ongoing]
This illness requires leadership – but it is like seeking nominations for the reins of an anarchist party; it goes against the foundations of our being to lead, and we don't necessarily work well together as a collective.

[2016]
I wanted to plead with the news services that day to understand her legacy in mental health advocacy when they reported on her passing. I feared this would be overlooked because about a billion too many teenage boys jerked off to images of her in a gold bikini, but, for the most part, I was proven wrong. *WHO Magazine* – the weekly tabloid that is usually about the receding, or resurfacing, fat on Hollywood bodies – ran a cover story about her death with the headline 'Her Amazing Life'. Please note the absence of 'tragic' or 'crazy' or 'fucked up' in that description. The writers also went with 'colourful and complicated', which – well, whose life isn't colourful and complicated?

[2017]

Mostly though, through all of this, I am hopeful that over the coming years people will slowly discover her traces in this separate, parallel sphere of influence and that's where her life will take on new meaning for those who need it. If I say that 'Carrie Fisher was my mental health icon' what do I mean? Part of it is the fact of saying it at all – the idea of there being such a thing as a mental health icon, or a mental health hero – feels like a relatively new concept, and it's not just in the phrasing. As stigma around mental ill health recedes, advocates can emerge more freely. Fisher came from a place of intense privilege in order to speak out at all, and a spotlight was trained on her from early on, the stage already built, but to state as much is not to take away from her achievements in that particular arena.

Fisher has left us with so many leads as to how to handle the disorder and care for each other. She has left us with a significant body of literature on the subject, in the form of semi-autobiographical novels and memoirs; *Postcards from the Edge* and *Wishful Drinking* being the best examples of those respective forms of work. There are countless interviews on late-night talk shows. There are memes explaining her definitions of the illness. There are more than 2000 tweets; some of them in the most cryptic form, but nearly always entertaining. No one who experiences mania is likely to complain about a lack of productivity, although you can't assume that the disorder will make you naturally talented or your writing any good, as that's a dangerous qualitative game you don't want to play. Most astonishingly, just a month before her death, she published an advice column in the *Guardian* written to a young woman, newly diagnosed with bipolar, in which she wrote:

We have been given a challenging illness, and there is no other option than to meet those challenges. Think of it as an opportunity to be heroic – not 'I survived living in Mosul during an attack' heroic, but an emotional survival. An opportunity to be a good example to others who might share our disorder. That's why it's important to find a community – however small – of other bipolar people to share experiences and find comfort in the similarities … As your bipolar sister, I'll be watching. Now get out there and show me and you what you can do.

Most importantly, it would seem, she provided us with a way to reach out and talk to each other, a radical act for what is, almost by definition, an internalised and painfully isolating illness.

[2016–17]
I wrote most of what is contained in this little, informal missive on the morning of her death, before I decided to walk away from the thoughts and take some time by myself. I thought that Carrie would have wanted me to treat myself well on the overwhelming news of her passing and that there is really the heart of it for me. Forevermore somewhere in the back of my complex mind, I'll be thinking: I think Carrie would want me to treat myself that way.

[2003]
Suzanne Vale made her return in *The Best Awful*, a sequel to *Postcards from the Edge*. This novel is her most direct about Fisher's experiences with manic depression (including the

memoir). It is her best novel – fully formed, with a Bello-vian pace and wit. If it had been written by a man (and non-celebrity), it likely would have been received better, and would not have been so unkindly reviewed. Rachel Cooke, a critic for the *Guardian*, reviewed *The Best Awful* on its release. In a deflating tone, Cooke pressed her case:

> *The Best Awful*, whose unlikely Hollywood ending I won't spoil, suffers from a literary version of the bipolar disorder that so cripples its heroine (and – surprise – its author, who requires two dozen pills a day to control the condition). When it is good, it is ... well ... fine; when it is bad, which is too often, it is absolutely bloody awful, so toxically terrible you feel like rushing out of doors and burying it at the bottom of the garden.

That Cooke is deliberately evoking the swings of a mood disorder to describe her critical reaction to the book points towards a kind of stigma of its own. She writes:

> In fictional terms, there are few things so boring as a nervous breakdown (unless we are talking Salinger), and the one described in such breathless detail in *The Best Awful* ranks with the work of Elizabeth Wurtzel when it comes to tedium.

This seems lazy, and, worse, kind of dangerous – weapon-ising an illness for the sake of critical point scoring. I count it as a betrayal.

[2011]

Fisher's 2011 memoir *Shockaholic* contains a long meandering essay about her friendship with Michael Jackson. Fisher follows the strange textures of his existence, and then his untimely death. There are similarities in their lives, namely coming to fame early – she was there from her first breath – and both having become so visually iconic with their outlandish costumes, whether onscreen or in real life. Fisher wrings a fine line out of the friendship: 'My reality – my *sur*-reality has set up housekeeping on my nerves.' In her short book *On Michael Jackson*, the cultural critic Margo Jefferson concludes her exploration of the psyche of pop music's greatest enigma by citing Kay Redfield Jamison:

> Within just three paragraphs of her book *An Unquiet Mind: A Memoir of Moods and Madness*, the psychiatrist and manic-depressive Kay Redfield Jamison uses three different terms: 'mental illness', 'madness' and 'abnormal mental states and behaviour'. She knows that unstable states of being unnerve people and create unstable language. 'Mental illness' may sound patronizing, but at least it's clinical; 'madness' in the wrong mouth amounts to a stigma. So, how do people talk about conditions, states of being, that wrench, confuse, disgust and scare them? People take refuge in the vernacular: it offers a form of mastery. Inventive. Brutally frank or slyly euphemistic …

[2017]

Following her death, and thinking of her as a mental health icon, a friend, with whom I share a similar camp sense of humour and this illness, came to call Fisher 'Mama'.

[1987]

From *Postcards from the Edge*: 'Sometimes I don't think I was made with reality in mind.'

[2017]

And now the end is clear: as I finish work on this book, walking around the city in a daze, there are images of Carrie all around – the ubiquitous marketing machine promoting *Star Wars: The Last Jedi* have made her, and her co-stars, inescapable – and that is no bad thing. It reminds me of the year before and how much she is still part of our culture. Travelling down to Melbourne for a funeral, I walk past the IMAX theatre, where a large-scale poster is strung on a frame that juts tall into the sky. I can isolate that image on my phone and take a photo. She is looking down on the city surrounds. The Disney reworking of the *Star Wars* films has involved the original cast, and it is hard imagining any other actor of Fisher's age – or Mark Hamill's for that matter – being used so prominently to promote such an expensive project. I go to see the film at a 7 a.m. screening back in Sydney, and watch with curiosity as to how the filmmakers will handle her departure. In an early, yet climactic, battle scene, Fisher's General Leia is blown into empty space – and the audience gasps, 'They killed her off' – but then, floating against a black backdrop, her hand moves and she shows signs of life. She turns and begins to float through space, heading back to her ship. It is a weird and eerie moment in an otherwise conventional action film, and one hopes that they knew they could only create such a moment for her. There's a sense of rightness in the world in watching that moment, and although it is a fiction, it represents something of her legacy and life, an ability to recover and come back again and again. The film will be debated and dissected for years to come, but her life will be decoded for many, many more, for those who know something of what it is like to float through black eternal space and, somehow, return.

TWO
LIVES

10

THIS IS ALL TO SAY THAT I DO NOT KNOW THE STORY AT ALL

1 One of the very first questions you are asked when a psychiatrist is fumbling towards a 'bipolar' diagnosis relates to family history. This is a nod towards the genetic, hereditary nature of the disease, but also a narrative framing device. Who? When? What? How? Why? The line is traceable. And I had it on both sides – it was tangible, and the record was real. One must reckon with this. Mine pointed in two directions – paternal and maternal – a bad-luck genetic gamble that came up 'manic' on receipt. This is all just history repeating itself. This is all to say that I had two relatives in my family tree – on either side – who had experienced madness, and potentially mania, of some form during their lifetimes. Both had been dead for decades by the time I was born. I have been written into existence by those who came before me. My genetic code contains their flaws – theirs are mine, mine theirs. Are we in this together?

2 As a child, I was, to put it mildly, obsessed with Walter Murch's *Return to Oz*, the unexpected 1985 sequel to the MGM classic musical. Murch – who remains best known as Francis Ford Coppola's go-to editor on films like

The Conversation and *Apocalypse Now* – hardly seemed an obvious choice to direct the sequel, which forgoes musical numbers for a deeper engagement with the mythology of L Frank Baum's bizarro series beyond the original novel. The film flopped on release in the cinemas, barely earning back half its budget, which was largely attributed to its inappropriate-for-children dark edges. I watched it over and over on VHS when it hit video stores, perhaps too young. The film, released in my year of birth, captured my childhood imagination like no other. The villainous henchmen in the film – the Wheelers – inspired me to go around the house holding a rolling pin between my two hands, using it to wheel across the linoleum floors. I would try to screw people's heads off like the bad witch Mombi.

When it was first put on for me, however, my grandparents were in the room, watching along. My grandfather left the room deeply upset somewhere within the first act. The film opens on the familiar Kansas farmhouse, where the young Dorothy Gale lives following the destructive tornado that has put her family's welfare in jeopardy. She's disturbed, and this, along with her constant retelling of the fantastical stories of 'Oz', has her Aunt Em and Uncle Henry deeply concerned. In the first film the explanation for Oz is found in the fact that Dorothy is dreaming, combined with likely trauma to the head from the tornado, which supposedly transports her to the imagined city. But in *Return to Oz*, and according to Aunt Em, Dorothy is having trouble sleeping. So, instead, she is lying awake, having wide-eyed lucid dreams about her memories of Oz.

They chance upon an advertisement in the newspaper which promises an 'electrical cure' and, with a loan from another aunt, take Dorothy away for treatment. The treatment, of course, is a primitive form of electroconvulsive therapy, or ECT.

My grandfather left the room in distress because his mother, Lily May Twyford, had been admitted to the psychiatric hospital in Callan Park and was given the same treatment in his youth. He never spoke of the matter. Who knew a children's film would elicit such a response?

In thinking about writing this book, I tried to follow leads to find out the truth – Callan Park burnt many of their patient records in the 1970s – but I kept coming back to the uncomfortable fact that I didn't know what happened.

The hospital operated in Rozelle under the name The Callan Park Hospital for the Insane until 1914. Then it became the Callan Park Mental Hospital until 1976, when it was finally shortened to Callan Park Hospital. I would, eventually, come to work next door at the NSW Writers' Centre. The office window would look out onto the grounds of the hospital, which was now used for the Sydney College of the Arts. Ghosts surely roamed about, but I never saw them on my lunch breaks.

3 Let the dead lie, and all that. The only information I could prise out of my relatives about Lily was that she was hospitalised for 'hysteria' following a complicated hysterectomy. This felt like shorthand for something else entirely – smoke and mirrors. But I couldn't find records to prove otherwise. I didn't know the truth, and many people with a hereditary mental illness do not know this either. If this feels underwritten and fleeting, I have to ask, 'Have I not done the work, not performed my job?' That's likely to assume I didn't

set myself this task. There are things you simply can't know and dead ends truly are dead in some cases. To not go out and find what really happened and to simply say, 'I do not know' is its own kind of truth. Regardless, I wish to leave the question quietly hanging in the air.

4 And, anyway, this is all to say that I do not know the story at all.

5 When my paternal grandmother was dying – raging as cancer laid waste to her thin frame, although she still managed to do her phone banking the day before she slipped into her final coma – her family came together at her small, modest home two hours north of Sydney to help her through the final days and to support each other. She was a true matriarch who controlled the family's emotional states for decades and convinced most of us to become nudists, to strip down in approved public places. She also conned everyone into practising reiki for a couple of decades as well as convincing us to do yoga. I didn't mind the yoga, and still occasionally repeat some of the stretches, but all of this bodily movement and her holistic approach hid her brilliant mind control strategies. She drove her children and grandchildren mad, and there was a feral edge to all of us in the end.

As when anyone dies, greedy eyes start laying claim to useless objects around the house. My grandmother was a painter and we were all mentally dividing up her personal collection as she shuffled from bed to bathroom, her legs swollen, waterlogged, as her organs shut down.

There was a factional concern for the artistic work of her long-dead brother, Laurence Tognetti – who this piece is really supposed to be about. Laurence was a painter too, but he was dead by 1950, so he didn't leave behind the largest body of work. The paintings were scattered between family members and it was hard to pull them all together. As my grandmother lay dying in the room next door, the faction, gathered, started to espouse theories that there were works hidden in the house and that we needed to find them. The stresses of dealing with nearby death and the uncertainty of the future of this family unit sent each individual, and each faction, around the bend. This lust for his paintings could have just been an outlet for some of the brewing madness and fear. I forgive the faction, of course, for that.

This is all a way, however, of framing the perceived value of Laurence Tognetti's work within my family. Emotions run high. There is a feeling that he is the lost genius of our line-age, his work is culturally significant and of the highest artistic order. Of course, none of that is true. His paintings, all nas-cent and derivative, have no real market value and never will. There will be no renaissance of interest in him, because there was never any interest in the first place. It didn't help that he shot himself in the head – and that he did it so far from home in Papua New Guinea just distanced him further from his roots.

6 I had seen one of Laurence's artworks before. The painting was hanging in my aunt's hallway; beneath it was a photograph of the painter himself in military uniform. It was a painting I knew only in passing – I walked past it quite a bit, but had never really stopped to give it very much

attention, nor had I, growing up, given much attention to the painter himself. He was long dead by the time I was born; there were more than thirty years between his death and my birth. The painting doesn't really speak to me on its own: it is a precise swirling of colour and abstract shape, crafted in a cool blue register, with warm bursts of yellow, like the light breaking through in religious paintings. The image folds in on itself and the painting can't quite carry the weight of its own abstraction. Taken with the story of its creator, however, it suddenly carries more meaning.

This might be why my aunt put the photograph of the painter so very close to it – a domestic curatorial quirk, necessary to give the work its due import. A field of shapes, folding in on themselves, as if in a state of several minor implosions. It looks to me like a Frank Hinder knock-off – even seeming to directly lift exact shapes from that well-known Sydney-born, American-trained modernist. His paintings were derivative, but this was likely because he was only ever a student, albeit a very talented one. He never made it past student stage because he never made it past the age of twenty-seven and much of his short life was spent in the military, serving in the Second World War. He didn't die in the war though.

Death configures us all in the abstract. Details of our lives, rendered secondhand, have little to do with reality. Be warned, your life can become rumour, as his did. But there were some known facts.

7 Laurence James Tognetti was born in Balmain, Sydney in 1923. The Tognetti family had emigrated to Australia from Switzerland at the turn of the twentieth

century. They landed in Dubbo, of all places likely chasing the Gold Rush. Why anyone would trade the altitudes of Switzerland for the flat expanse of regional plains that surround Dubbo is beyond me. The growing family then traded Dubbo for Leichhardt in Sydney, where they opened a number of small businesses and put into action one illegal distillery. It seemed to be a family of ratbags – the illegal distillery, and its discovery, made the pages of the *Sydney Morning Herald* – but when the Depression hit, and the businesses were closed, that sense of fun was dampened. The family were moved to the slums of Glebe, and the coming war saw the two eldest sons sent to far-flung stations to serve – Laurence to Papua New Guinea, his brother Gordon to Crete.

During my second mania, I visited my cousin, the violinist and artistic director of the Australian Chamber Orchestra, Richard Tognetti, in the hope of writing a portrait of him for a newspaper – the photographer Weeds was in tow to take portrait shots – but it never came to fruition. Over lunch, we talked about many things, but the whole time I was thinking how, in many ways, Richard – listed by the National Trust of Australia as one of the country's 100 National Living Treasures – was Laurence's promise made good. I brought up Laurence and what I had discovered and was surprised to learn that Richard hadn't heard of his uncle's fate. The suppression of the story is the story in its own way.

8 The spelling of his name is inconsistent across official documents, going between Lawrence and Laurence – a sign of inconsistencies to come. In a letter written to his mother from Papua New Guinea, he gave a possible sign of

as to why: 'I hope you were not too confused when my friend asked for "Jim" – you see I have always had a bit of an aversion to Laurence – at least in the army – because if there is more than one syllable in your name everyone promptly forgets and you usually get some other nickname which may not sound too good and is usually offensive, so you will no doubt appreciate why I changed it.'

9 I discovered a small parcel of Laurence's letters in my parents' house, containing this letter to his mother and many others addressed to his sister, my grandmother, Irene, with whom he appeared to have a close relationship, filled with sibling teasing and love. I quote them here to impart a sense of his character, and the conditions under which he lived during the war. They are complete in themselves, but there must be others out there that paint a fuller picture of his mind at the time. I quote a single letter here, in full, and offer some parts from others, simply to give you a picture of his great sense of humour, and his affection for his sister:

LJ Tognetti
AAM 6 atl
38 Aust Workers Bay
Australia
13.10.44

Dear Irene,

Last Sunday Frank and I met some AMWAS down at the beach and they invited us up to the hospital to their mess. It was very nice to have some female company for a change – we told them we hadn't seen a white woman for about two years and they took pity on us, it was rather hard trying to meet them as there is a lot of hungry wolves (male) prowling around up here.

I will just explain the procedure if you wish to take one to the pictures – first of all you have to see the sergeant in charge of the AMWAS and she examines you with a suspicious look in her eyes, and finds out all your family history, and when you get over this ordeal you have to sign for her (like a negotiated parcel) so you see they take no chances.

On Thursday we had an inter-unit game of football and I was kept busy carrying the ladies off the field, it's hot enough, without indulging in any strenuous exercise, and I had a big sick headache the next morning.

We found a small tree python curled up, enjoying a snooze in the rafters of the RAP, so after rendering him innocuous with some boiling water I sliced his head off with my scalpel and put him under the sergeant major's bed – but he failed to see the humour of it.

Well that is all for the present.

Lots of love
Laurence

P.S. Thanks a lot for the medical dictionary and I would be very pleased if you could send me up some drawing pencils.

Two charcoal
Two soft
One hard

I am still looking forward to the cakes. I hope the
censors haven't eaten it.

[No date]
A humorous though painful incident occurred at the
concert down the road last night. The chap on the
stage was doing the hangman's act and it was hardly
successful. He got four big heft fellows from the
audience, tied some rope round his neck and gave a
piece of rope to the four chaps and told them to pull –
and they did – first of all his tongue poked out, then
his eyes popped out, then he popped over – they almost
choked him.

3.1.45

Christmas and the New Year has [sic] passed without
a great deal of excitement up here. A couple of my
friends sat up until about 1 o'clock on New Year's Eve
drinking malted milk – but I failed to see the fun of
it. Still, we really cannot complain. We did very wll
considering – I only hope Gordon did as well – but I
don't think the Germans are altogether imbibed with
the Christmas spirit. I was just interrupted in writing
by a chap who brought in an eel which he caught down

the creek, so tomorrow we will have it for breakfast –
they are quite palatable when cooked properly, lately
the boys have been catching quite a number of them
and also some fish. The only trouble however is when
we go for a swim we expect the eels to but [sic] us on
the toes.

3.1.45

I suppose you have made a New Years [sic] resolution
not to go out more than six nights a week.

3.1.45

Every morning the Medical Officer visits the RAP to
examine the long suffering sick parade … He is a very
nice chap but he makes me listen very attentively to the
patients [sic] complaints (which are usually many and
varied) as afterwards I have to diagnose the complaint
and I am more often wrong than right. I finish up
with a complicated medical lecture, but it very [sic]
interesting and enlightening.

10 Reading the letters now, how I long for an easier, more
literal connection in all of this. A missive explaining
his exact state of mind: 'Dear Irene, I am writing to you as

I fear I am suffering *folie à double forme*, or perhaps it is *folie circulaire*! I guess they would call it manic depression back home. Oh well, suppose it's to the asylum, or otherwise death, for me! Tell your future grandson he can write whatever he wants about my life, and that he is free to quote from my letters at will.'

11 Late in the game, my great uncle, still kicking, sent me a letter from Laurence to my grandfather – his best friend, Charles Moore, a man who would become his brother-in-law, after my grandmother's first marriage broke down three years after Laurence's death. The letter is covered in cartoon heads – one screaming 'Moore for President!' another 'Less for Moore!' The letter is written from Laurence's fictitious 'palatial office'. As he surveys 'the vast organisation I am the omnipresent director of' he is hit by a 'wave of nostalgia … I remember the unfortunate friends who had not the ruthless determination to attain the colossal heights I have transcended. I remember my poor old friend Charles sweating his wasted emaciated body and soul (if any) …' The letter – one that echoes Spike Milligan's own cartoon-infested correspondence – reminds me of my own sense of humour and life, surely inherited from this lineage, and makes me feel close to a man impossible to meet.

12 Laurence returned home, deeply affected by the war and what he had seen there. He struggled to hold down a steady job. He saved a three-year-old girl from drowning, and the story made the papers. He wandered; he

was lost, according to others. He had movie-star good looks according to his brother. He was loved, but he was lost; so lost. So, he returned to Papua New Guinea and finished the job that the war hadn't: he killed himself. The idea of returning to the site of conflict to perform this haunts me. It seems too apt. And the story isn't straight. There was no diagnosis of mental illness. And the details have been blurred by time and fumbled mistellings.

His mother, in frail health, was told that he had been hit, and killed, by a bus. But if this was just a white lie to an elderly woman, could it be true too in a way? He could have stepped out in front of a bus to kill himself. The bus is just a story, but fictions have their truths, and white lies have their place. History is written with gentle lies. The one truth – he was dead – was all that counted in the end.

One relative commented that he believed that Laurence had been playing Russian roulette when he shot himself. Graham Greene, another manic depressive, was known to play the game too. There is no game with higher stakes.

I am no historian. I fumble with the facts and stumble with the rules of this telling. I didn't do all the research I could have. The original pitch for this book was to travel to PNG and follow the leads into Laurence Tognetti's death – what a stunning thriller! What intrigue! But I didn't have the resources, nor the nerve. Give me more time, and I'll deliver the goods. Also, such travel would put my own mental health at risk, surely.

His suffering and death could very easily be put down to PTSD from the war. What did he see? Piles of bodies, dead friends; and he had a brother to worry about in a POW camp in Germany. So was this a madness specific to war, or just a general mania, embedded in his genetic materials, and passed on to mine?

13 This is all to say that I do not know the story at all.

A
LIFE

11

THE RAPIDS: A CODA IN CUTS

A Yoyo from Hell

The last time I was in it, I knew I was in it. This was different from the other times, when I was in it, but I did not know that I was in it. We looked up hospital beds in private clinics, but at $2000 a night, we could not afford to admit me. So, we rented a serviced apartment for a week at half the cost, and I started smoking and watching movies. I was manic, so I was spending too much money, buying loose-fitting t-shirts and DVDs. There was conflict in the background and my head thrummed with pain from it, and my moods were swinging out of control. It was the first time I experienced a mixed state, up and down like a demented yoyo from hell. That yoyo had more string to it than I realised.

LOL/SOS

During my second sustained manic episode, I decided to get a tattoo for the first time. A lasting marker on my skin of my time spent out of my mind. Fortunately, it turned out to be tasteful, and, staring at it on my arm now, remains meaningful. A good friend sent me a picture from a small Amsterdam-based design collective named *metahaven*. The image was described as 'A definition of now' and was laid out as follows:

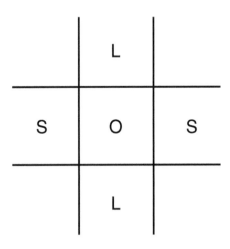

Immediately, I knew, almost instinctually, that I wanted the image on my skin. I emailed around and found a tattoo artist who could come over to my house and for $100 put this thing on my arm permanently. With this new skin, Weeds and I went walking through bush scrub in Canberra to get some shots. We walked down to the cool waters of the Kambah Pool, and Weeds directed me to lie about, taking shots with his cool, cool camera. He sent me onto a rock poking out of the water and directed me to step back. I tripped and fell, grabbing onto a tree, which grazed my arm. The tattoo was cut up, and despite the searing pain, I couldn't help but laugh. LOL featured a gash down the centre of the tic-tac-toe game inked on my skin. We drove to a cemetery after that to visit my cousin's grave as we prepared to drive out of Canberra for good. I sat at the quiet site – thirteen years after his death from a brain aneurism at the age of seventeen – and bawled.

LOL-well

In her long, loving exploration of the life of one of America's most iconic poets, *Robert Lowell: Setting the River on Fire*, Kay Redfield Jamison dives into Lowell's lifelong struggle with manic depression. The book – part biography, part literary study, part personalised medical history – comes with the subtitle *A Study of Genius, Mania, and Character*. To craft a portrait of Lowell's character, Redfield Jamison combs through letters between Lowell and his contemporaries, and in particular his wife Elizabeth Hardwick. Mania, Lowell had mused, was an 'extremity, for one's friends, depression an illness of oneself'.

There is always desperation in the hope that this will be the last of the manias. Robert Lowell struggled with this hope – and the sense of its futility – towards the end of his life. Redfield Jamison locates some of his dialogues in relation to this. He wrote to Frank Bidart, after leaving hospital again, 'I am weighed down by the new frequency of attacks. How can one function, if one is regularly sick. [sic] Shades of the future prison'. He told the Australian artist Sidney Nolan, 'I've been sixteen times on my knees. I've got up sixteen times. But if one day I don't get up, I don't mind.'

To a young lover, he said, 'If I had a button I'd switch myself off. The show's been going on too long.'

Soundtrack

One of the most notable features of mania is a high level of irritability – of which I possibly have not written enough, but it is rather irritating to even think back on it – and so noises, smells and the general presence of others are enough to set you off. I believe that senses are heightened during this time. Music seeps into your ears with more clarity and assumed meaning. So there were soundtracks to my manias – songs which I would listen to over and over again – which I believed spoke directly to me. It's like being a teenager again. Here is a list of songs that embedded into my consciousness while manic (and listening to them now, they have the Proustian quality of not only recalling memory, but awakening certain emotions of the time in which I listened to them):

[2008]

Kes Band, 'Gentle Elf'

The voice of Karl Scullin (aka Kes) is a strange wonder – high but not a falsetto, scratchy but soothing. This song was discovered through a Christmas compilation from a Melbourne-based indie record company, the CD of which I stole from a JB Hi-Fi in the midst of a mania-induced kleptomanic spree.

Sly Hats, 'Liquorice Nights'

Again, the pull towards Melbourne was strong, facilitated by listening to bands from there. See also: Birth Glow, Pikelet et al. These albums might have been stolen too.

Yo La Tengo, 'Autumn Sweater' (Kevin Shields remix)

It is important to distinguish that this was the remix by Kevin Shields, the reclusive genius frontman of Irish shoegaze icons My Bloody Valentine. This heady mix was on repeat as I screamed towards Melbourne.

[2015]

Justin Bieber, 'Sorry'

This might be the clearest indication that this was the strongest of my manias – unabashed, indulgent pop suddenly took over my headphones/rental car speakers, and I was lost in the wash that resulted.

The Chills, 'Warm Waveform'

Music is there to obsess over but how many times can you listen to the one song? A lot if mania has anything to do with it.

Drake, 'Headlines'

Drizzy gave me the confidence I already had inside me, in surplus. Sometimes listening to a song can be very bad for you indeed. I wanted to burn things.

Grimes, 'California'

I've said before that California is a dangerous site of mania for me. This propulsive song represented that.

Hans Zimmer, 'Mountains'

Zimmer's soundtrack to Christopher Nolan's underrated space melodrama *Interstellar* is all enveloping when listened to on headphones. I remember taking my laptop down to the beach, listening to 'Mountains' and feeling as if I was travelling through space and time (which, technically, of course we are). It was like being on LSD without ever having to bother with putting the tab on your tongue.

[2017]

I can't remember much from this episode, my memory is wrecked, my iTunes deleted to make space on my hard drive and anyway what is the point of this – if you tracked down these songs, or I gave them to you as a mixtape and you listened to them, what would they even sound like to you? They couldn't possibly evoke my mania for you. I do remember I was listening to a lot of New Order – across the catalogue, but particularly late-era live remixes of earlier work – if that helps at all. Do remixes soothe a manic mind with their variations?

Begin Again

I had become, at the mid-point of that fast summer, an increasingly fidgety person, prone to pacing the house and, occasionally, jogging around it in a dog-legged dash. I had extra energy that I needed to rid myself of. It wouldn't just disappear, and nothing around me moved at the same speed I was going at. The only thing that would settle me down was watching tennis on the television. It was hard to say what about tennis created this soothing effect. Perhaps it was the perpetual back and forth of the ball, which created a hypnotic rhythm. This had variations and breaks, but for the most part there was the routine thwack of the ball meeting the racquet and a sigh or grunt from the player. These rough beats were reproduced in my head and steadied everything. It was better than drinking myself to sleep – an option that was not fully on the table after a recent bout of alcohol intolerance – and as the games often went late and were sometimes repeated early in the morning, they kept me calm at a time when my fidgeting felt out of control. January meant that there was plenty of tennis on the TV, with the Australian Open taking up most of the prime time of one of the commercial channels. I would stay awake after the games, walking around my lounge room near Newcastle, thinking about what it would be like to watch the matches in the arena down in Melbourne.

It was way past midnight, after a particularly emotional game – Roger Federer cried as he clutched the spoils of victory – when I decided to turn speculation into action: it was possible to get down to Melbourne in time for the next match. I packed the few basics I thought I would need and a sleeping bag into the boot of my rusting, somewhat troubled 1987 Holden Vacationer and left my home on the Central Coast – what they call the 'taint between the dick and balls of Sydney and Newcastle' – at 4 a.m. The only vehicles on the road were garbage trucks and long-haul eighteen-wheelers. I got into the spirit of elite sports and tried to break my personal best in driving speed. Hooning down the F3, I did 140 km/h for sneaky stretches of the twelve hours, keeping an eye out for cop cars. I shot through Sydney by the time the sun showed itself. I got lost on the south coast and ended up on the edge of a ditch, eating untoasted pop tarts straight from the box.

I had a micro-sleep as I finally drove into Melbourne, fourteen hours of driving later. I had only closed my eyes for a fraction of a second, but it caused me to swerve slightly off the road just before I came onto Sydney Road. I booked into a central hostel, took the small steel lift up to the TV room and sat in front of a 36-inch widescreen. I'd come all the way to Melbourne to watch the tennis, as on arrival, I had lost all desire to go anywhere near Rod Laver Arena. I could have watched the games at home, but convinced myself that it was different watching it on TV in Melbourne, closer to the actual events. I fell asleep in front of the communal TV in my underwear that night after watching pre-game, game and post-game analysis. When I woke up, my bank cards were gone and I had no money for another night at the hostel, so it was time to go home. I was still fidgety enough to drive back to Sydney twenty-four hours after arriving in Melbourne.

Breakdown

The car carked it just outside of the nation's capital at what should have been the rough halfway mark to home. The engine was over-heating – the oil temp light flashed red on the dashboard to tell me so, but that seemed less pertinent than the steam rising out of the bonnet. The acceleration was slow to respond. The road was stretching on but it looked like the car would not make it past the next bend of the Hume Highway. I slowed down and pulled over into a rest area, where families picnicked on brown benches and an elderly couple were staring at the sun. I opened the bonnet and checked the oil. I poured water into the place I had been shown; as it touched the hot metal inside it went off like a geyser. I stepped back and rushed to get more water from a leaking knee-high tap. I looked around to ask for help but all eyes were on sandwiches and cold cans of drink.

I had sweat on my brow, which dripped into the twisting black innards of the greasy engine as I did my best to revive it. The car had not committed suicide – the whole explosive situation was not its fault, and as much as I might have liked to, I didn't kick in the fender or smash the headlights with a raised foot or pound on the bonnet with clenched fists. The car was old and marked by death. I had not been treating it right. It had originally been lined up to be given to my cousin – my aunt was going to pass it on to him instead of trading it in to some used car lot, but he dropped dead from a bleeding brain before she had the chance. She gave me the car shortly after his funeral. I made a mess of the rear window by placing stickers for radio stations over it. My father called it 'John Boy' after my cousin, which I remember thinking was creepy at the time. I respected my father's naming rights, though. This was a dead boy's car and maybe an altar is what it should have been. I did all the things that my cousin would no longer be able to do in it, stopping short of having sex on the seats and smoking bongs in the back. I drove it, listening to songs on crappy tapes bought from the local supermarket; this felt like the best way I could pay my dues. The songs played through the single speaker that still worked – even it suffered the death rattles – but the sound was amazingly clear. I could hear every word.

That the car looked like it was on its last legs was upsetting, but there was a certain thrill when I managed to get back on the highway. It wasn't to last – there was only a kilometre or two of highway left before the car conked out for good.

I had to get out of the way of the murderous stream of traffic. The nearest turn-off was Yass. Making it to Canberra was out of the question. I turned in to a ditch and killed an already-dead engine. I got out and looked around. Nothing but yellowing grass and the exit to a highway I should have still been on.

The House Is Indifferent to Me

There was a fibro house at the corner and I went around the side, turned on a tap and drank from the mouth of a hose. I could hear the family inside as my cheeks filled with water hot from the sun. I needed to find a pay phone or someone who would lend me access to their line. I didn't feel like knocking on a random family's door. I slumped into the wet grass, and from this low point of view spied a bed and breakfast across the road.

I tried to find the reception of the main house, then went and knocked on the door of the dining hall, which was to the side in its own building. I went and called out at the house at the back, which I assumed to be the owner's residence. There was no 'vacant' sign but one might as well have been flickering over every part of the grounds. It was ghost-town quiet. I went to the back window of the main house and tore open the flyscreen. It made the sound of Velcro ripping – a sound I'd heard before, somewhere else – and I wanted to keep going once I had ripped all the way to the top because I liked the sound so much. I climbed up and through the window and put my feet down in a room decorated in an overly precious Victorian style. There were tea cosies on a dressing table and small packaged soaps on the pillows, dried potpourri beside the bed, starched white sheets folded on a rocking chair. There was no luggage in the room and it looked as if nothing had been moved for months.

I walked around the house and found four identical rooms and a shared living space with a TV and DVD player. There was no phone, though. I packed up some of the DVDs and put them in the back seat of the broken-down car, next to my hardback copy of Leonard Michaels' *Collected Stories* and about twenty other books, some of which I had bought from online bookstores and promptly forgotten to read, and others which I had stolen from the front of shops. (I had developed a technique of walking into a shop with a copy of a broadsheet newspaper and slipping a book into the paper, before walking through the store's sensors with the newspaper over my head.)

The dining hall seemed more likely to house a phone. I peered inside and saw one by the register. The windows and doors would not move for me. I got a rock from the garden bed and considered lobbing it through the double doors at the front, but thought about the noise and the family in their living room across the road. I imagined them dialling the police. Instead, I used it to smash a small side window. The glass shattered across the floor of the kitchen. I cut my hand as I climbed through the window. It wasn't a bad cut. I wrapped my hand with some tissues and tape and made myself a chocolate milkshake with syrup and milk from the fridge, in a tall yellow paper cup with a green palm tree design wrapped around it, and drank it down fast. I didn't really need any more energy than I already had, but the glucose gave me an extra kick to get through the whole drawn-out process of the break and enter. I had never used a cash register before, but it was fairly self-explanatory. I pressed one button and it opened itself up immediately. There were riches in the till – $100 notes – and I took them all, leaving the coins. I had no need for them. There were $50 notes too. I stuffed them into my pockets.

I went around to the other side of the counter and found a blackboard leaning against a table, on which the specials menu would have been written. I wiped it clean with my forearm and picked out a piece of coloured chalk from an ice-cream container. I got down on my knees and wrote my repentance:

I AM SORRY FOR DOING THIS. I AM VERY
POOR AND WOULD NEVER STEAL BUT I AM
IN A VERY BAD WAY. I AM SORRY.

That was pure bullshit, or to put it more gently, my fiction. I was not so poor and despite the cut hand I was not in such a bad way, or at least I did not feel bad. I felt quite good, looking around the empty dining hall; I had a new hang-out. I had access to food and books. There were only commercial fiction titles on the bookshelves, though, nothing I actually wanted to read – romance novels for weekend getaways. There was no real food in the industrial-sized freezers, either, just base ingredients and I did not feel as if I had time to cook. I walked down to Yass Junction instead, populated by a small strip of cafés and shops, and with my pockets filled with new cash I would have my pick of every menu. There was a simple-looking place and I went in and ordered a tuna salad, a large coffee, lemonade and carrot cake. The food was all orange, yellow and brown and this was somehow comforting, when it should have made me push the plate away and not touch the coffee. I had always eaten fast, with a fidgety foot scratching the other, but there seemed to be no swallowing here. I just absorbed the food. I bought some gum to get the sensation of chewing back.

I considered staying a night at a hotel a few doors down, but figured I better get out of town. I went into the mechanic's across the road and told them about my car, asking what could be done. Their books were filled for the rest of the week. That was no good to me.

I went back to the bed and breakfast and found that beside the owner's quarters was a car under a blue tarpaulin. I figured the keys for it would be somewhere in the house. I repeated the flyscreen rip and climbed through into a tight bathroom. Stepping out into the main bedroom, it felt odd standing in front of a stranger's bed. Near the door, on a table covered in keys, was more money. I took another $200. I went back outside and ripped the protective cover off the vehicle, revealing a red sports convertible. I opened the door, feeling relieved that I didn't have to smash glass to get in. I turned the key over. I turned the key again and again but it wouldn't start. It was lucky that it didn't, really. The car was a manual, which I didn't know how to drive. It seemed pointless to steal a car if you didn't know how to drive it. I imagined I would be able to learn in the backstreets of Yass – of which there were probably two – before hitting the highway and heading home. I'm not sure how I thought I was going to explain the car when I got there; how I had managed to trade in the dead Holden Vacationer for an MG Sports Car of the Year. It seemed to be that if the driver of such a car was not wearing a red leather jacket with sunglasses, then the whole driving experience would have been a waste, and I did not own a red leather jacket nor a pair of sunglasses at that point.

Glenrowan

I went into one of the unoccupied rooms and showered, ripping open the packeted soft white soap. The towels were white and clean. I lay on the sheets and called a taxi to make my getaway. Hit by a second wave of misguided creativity, I pulled a pen out from my back pocket and wrote a partial confession at the top of the sheet.

As I was close to the place where the bushranger Ned Kelly had been caught, and where I had just stolen a tank of petrol, I mused: 'Will *this* be my Glenrowan?'

Perhaps it was like wondering if the place would be my Waterloo. What a load of bullshit, looking back, but I was serious then. It wasn't any myth-making on my part. I *had* been pulled over by police earlier that day. Their blue and red lights flashed just as I hit the outskirts of Melbourne and made my move to get onto the Hume. I had been speeding out of the city like a hoon, looking forward to hitting the long country stretches, and right after stealing a tank of premium petrol. They didn't mention the stolen fuel, though – it was a simple case of speeding. They had caught me going at 114 km/h. Before putting on the brakes, I was almost certainly moving at 130 km/h. They asked for my licence. The only proof of identity I had was printed on the side of a packet of generic antidepressants, which I had not been taking. It should have been a flag for them, but they read the name and handed back the packet. I explained that my licence, as well as a bank card, had been stolen from a hostel I had been staying at. They did the routine check to make sure that the vehicle had not been stolen.

I watched them in the rear-view mirror as they talked on the radio. I was waiting for the cuffs, but they came over and handed me a ticket instead. The NSW plates must have made them think that I wasn't their problem. I imagined they thought I would get pulled up again once I was over state lines and it would be up to the NSW cops to deal with me.

Now in Yass, having broken into three separate buildings, I was expecting to see those blue and red lights flare up and flash again and when I heard the sound of footsteps coming from outside I imagined a can of tear gas coming through the windows. I wondered if the owner of the place could have a gun stored somewhere on site and whether he might go for it straight away on seeing the broken glass and the torn fly screens. The truth was that the illegality of all of these actions was extremely banal. I just wanted a hotel room and somewhere to sleep. Bonnie and Clyde and other bank robbers in crime films seemed to be acting out of boredom, but I couldn't help but feel my transgressions had come of necessity and the fact that, in the middle of Yass, I had nowhere else to go and nothing else to do. I was not trying to look bad-arse, because there was no one around, and because of that no one could see me.

The footsteps came around again and I got off the bed and lay down on the floor. I really did not want to be seen, but then I remembered ordering the taxi and went outside, just as the taxi driver was walking back to his cab to drive off.

'Sorry', I said. 'I was just saying goodbye to my grandparents. They're both almost deaf, but they heard you out the front before I did.'

253

For whatever reason – the promise of money, most likely – the taxi driver bought the story. He repaid me with a story about his ex-wife and how she would not let him see his son.

'She thinks that the boy is property. He's not something you can divide. He is both her and me in one.'

The taxi started to feel like the cramped inside of a psychologist's office. I should have charged him for my time. From Yass to Canberra it was a $200 taxi ride. I paid with the money I'd taken from the cash register. He didn't say anything about the fact that I had $800 in notes on me. I booked into a cheap drive-thru hotel on the outskirts of the capital. I went up to my room, a concrete pod with the bare minimum of natural light, and laid the money out on the bed in front of me, like a gangster in some dumb movie. I slept fitfully, watching pay-per-view movies, until I came up with a plan to get home at last.

Glenrowan II

I really had to face the fact of what I had done when the owner of the bed and breakfast sent the sheets to me in a white Australia Post package months later. The question was still there: 'Will *this* be my Glenrowan?' Maybe it had proven true. I had been caught and had to face up to my crimes.

Twyford Rising

How tempting it is to try and find meaning in the fact that the novelist Jay Griffiths had opened her memoir, *Tristimania: A Diary of Manic Depression*, with the proposition that 'If I had to pick the moment when it all began, I'd have to choose the afternoon at Twyford Down.' It was as if the universe had laid a trap. Twyford Down – an area of chalk downland in Winchester – had been the site of protest against a major motorway. Badges had been distributed to activists with the slogan 'Twyford Rising' printed on them. In my mind, I was screaming: 'Twyford Down/Twyford Rising!' Again, there is much temptation in these coincidences, and in a state of mania, I would latch onto them and project them onto anyone nearby. To make meaning is the gift and obligation of the writer, however, and to dismiss coincidence outright is risky for business.

Money

There is a chance to commodify the illness – the memoirs and the speaker circuits being the chief avenues for this pursuit of profit – and who shouldn't make a dollar out of pain? You can't keep that energy up – you hate that you can't keep that energy up, thank God you can't keep that energy up.

(Dis)associative

Let's say that mania is a dissociative state of mind, and yet, equally, that same mind, in that state, operates in a hyper-associative manner. Everything is connected, or has the possibility to be connected. I hope I have gone some way to proving this fact within this book, somewhere.

Crank

Looking back at the book made me consider what other arte-facts of the culture might have swung me in this direction. They certainly influenced the way I talked about mental illness. In an early psychology session, when asked if there was a history of mental ill health in my family, I started with my great-uncle: 'He's a crank.' Of course, he wasn't a confirmed case. He was just eccentric and he had no known diagnosis related to what I was going through. There were better exam-ples at hand but I thought it was important to bring him up for some reason. 'Crank?' the psychologist asked, confused. I had been reading too much Bellow, and so my language was out of date, and pitched far too high. There was a film out called *Crank* in which an assassin is poisoned and must keep his adrenalin 'cranking' to keep himself alive. Perhaps she thought I had seen that.

Language continued to confuse. In one session I said that I had, late one night, 'shot up in bed'. What I meant was shot upright, sitting suddenly after waking in fright, but the psy-chologist wanted to refer me to specialised drug counselling at the end of the session, which caused me great confusion.

Cycles

These depressions weren't straight in their direction. They didn't all go downward. At times they could be described as hysterical. I would run around the house umpteen times trying to escape my own moods. If I could only get ahead of myself, I would outrun them. I would cycle through bushlands, lacerat-ing myself for my poor state as fast as the wheels were turning. They involved personal grievances blown out of proportion.

Rental Cars

After ending up in Byron Bay, following being flown to Port Douglas for a ridiculous gig interviewing an author at a beach-side resort, there was a complex negotiation with a rental car company in order to get back home. After I declined to return the car to the place where I hired it, they wanted me to return it to nearby Coffs Harbour. I was gone though – both with the car, and in my mind. I was bolting back home, driving through the night. In the early hours of the morning, I pulled over into a service station and bought a large bottle of Pepsi, which I drank nearly whole. Taking off from the service station, I could feel my eyes growing weary. As I sped towards home, I could see flames – in the lane going in the other direction, a car was alight in the middle of the highway. It burnt brightly for a brief moment in my eye line, and then on the periphery, and then was gone. Had I gone mad? I was using my iPhone as a Dictaphone and improvising large grabs of a novel, then a play, then a rant involving aggrieved other parties. I lost all my money driving rental cars, not asking what they cost, and I was broke by the time I returned it, no longer able to afford to drive any car, ever.

Camera

In Oaxaca, Mexico, in a small musty hostel room, fighting, unexpectedly, with my travelling companion, I screamed and tore my shirt off my chest, and buttons scattered everywhere. I was out of breath, and suddenly without a shirt to wear out to the *zócalo*. Later that day, in another public square, outside of town, I smashed a digital camera on the ground under the shade of a 200-year-old tree.

I Have Worn Sunglasses

In his essay 'I Have Never Worn Sunglasses', the novelist Gerald Murnane talks about the things he hasn't done, chief amongst them the titular confession of never having worn sunglasses. I am the opposite – I have always worn sunglasses, not in reality but in my mind; I have always conceived of myself wearing sunglasses and have, for a long time, been searching out the perfect pair. At the end of that trip, I ended up with a very good pair – designed and made in Los Angeles, the city of my mania dreams (it is lucky I never have any money because I would invariably end up wasting it on flights to LA that I would never take) – with these gold-hued plastic round frames of the exact style I had long aspired to but had never been able to achieve. I've misplaced them for the moment (sunglasses aren't really sunglasses until they've been misplaced for a time), but I think about them all the time. So, because these were purchased during a period of mania, should I give them up? They seem to be a marker of that time; there was logic in the decision – good sunglasses are an investment, of which everyone needs a pair (the price was a little steep, but I was convinced they would reap dividends of some kind). I keep coming back to it: if I had it together enough to buy these sunglasses, did it mean I was experiencing mania at all?

Cooking

During most of my manic episodes, I have become obsessed with the art of cooking – the stranger the recipe the better. During my last mania, the most obvious outward sign in its early stages was the fact that I cooked a *timpano* for a friend's

Christmas party, inspired by the 1996 masterpiece *Big Night*, co-starring and co-directed by the eternally charming Stanley Tucci. Timpano is a monstrous dish of boiled eggs, cheese, meatballs, salami and pasta, all encased in a giant sheet of more pasta. I was too embarrassed to serve it, and walked out of the room when it was cut open to reveal the excessive cross-section. In my second manic episode, I got it in my head to make a beachscape as a dessert for friends. It was wildly, overly ambitious – dehydrated mango for sand, dill for sea-weed, yoghurt ice-cream for sea foam, candied jalapenos and lime slices, rum-soaked pineapple, and, inexplicably, inedible coconut husks, the serving plate surrounded by large shells – and this just might have been the clearest physical indicator that I was completely out of it. Things were simpler in my first manic episode, when the cooking urge came down to a gnawing need to make a kangaroo pie. I turned on the stove-top and got a heavy-bottom pan. In went diced onion and garlic. I fried off the meat. Kangaroo is tough and gamey if you overcook it, but I thought slow-cooking it in a pot might braise it enough to make it soft. Tomatoes and red wine for the gravy. Bay leaves and oregano added late in the mix. The sauce simmered on the stovetop and I transferred it to a white crockery pot, covering it with layers of filo pastry. I looked out the window as I placed the pie in the oven, and imagined mountains and going to the refrigerator to drink a glass of milk for an old high-school friend who had strange ideas too.

Kangaroo Milk

Henry, a sorta friend from high school, wasn't quite so far gone as I, but there were signs. I only have one really vivid memory of him. In the middle of one of our Modern History classes, focusing on the economic struggles of various nations during the Second World War, Henry had suggested we all move to the 'mountains' for a few months and milk kangaroos for foodstuffs. This, he said, would save both the environment and the economy. Everyone had laughed, including the stern teacher, and because Henry wasn't laughing with us, it was hard to tell if he was serious or joking, whether he was upset that we had dared laugh at the suggestion or whether he was basking in the glow of a successful joke. Comedians are hard to read.

'Yeah, and we could ride kangaroos around – that way we wouldn't use any fucking petrol,' one of the crueller kids in the class called out.

Where did this kangaroo idea come from?

There were rumours going around school that Henry was a manic depressive. I had never heard those two words put together before. I would not know that the words could be clinically joined as bipolar until they were pointed my way years later. This wasn't right. I was not like him. I didn't need to ask for help. I did my homework and stayed away from those dug-out druggie holes behind the basketball courts and I never, ever owned a skateboard and there was no way that I thought kangaroos could be milked and I wasn't even sure you could drink that stuff.

Henry's kangaroo obsession, however, caught up with me when I was in the middle of the most intense of my hypomanic swings. I adapted the theory, walking around the house, telling everyone I was going to cook a kangaroo pie. This did not seem so strange to me. Kangaroo was now widely available in supermarkets across the country. I had had wallaby – not available in supermarkets – on a pizza in Tasmania during the inaugural MOFO. My father had once had horse meat on a pizza when he was in Japan. But my parents and others I told about this recipe plan thought the idea of kangaroo pie was extremely off-colour. It seems socially acceptable to put whatever the hell you like on top of a pizza, but burying strange meats in a pie makes the food dark and ominous, as if you are intentionally hiding the offending matter under the lid of pastry.

Cop-out

This was the one disjuncture in my personality that I could never reconcile during my manics – that I had been edged towards reckless criminality. It was 'uncharacteristic' and one hopes that it is not a cop-out to claim it as such.

A Count

Looking at the index of *The Letters of Robert Lowell*, I despaired, staring at this run of page numbers:

> manic-depression, xi–xviii, xxviii, xxx, 144, 145, 151, 157, 160, 167, 235–39, 282, 288, 295, 308, 310, 315–19, 321, 322, 332, 340–41, 346–47, 351, 354, 379, 390, 444, 460, 465, 483, 521, 528–29, 552, 643, 645, 650, 667

And the numbers accumulated into a life! These were just mentions in the letters – scrawls, markers of, but not quite the lived experiences themselves – but for a moment, sitting in the lonely library, they looked as if they moved, became a life.

How many mentions would I so far have collected in dialogue with others if they were indexed in such a way? I remember reading somewhere that Spike Milligan had had nine or so breakdowns in his life. I imagined Lowell going longer, as if a footballer running for the end zone, taking the most points.

Stolen Books

I was reading *The Adventures of Augie March* and Roberto Bolaño's *The Savage Detectives* during these early manic episodes (it's funny that I could keep the attention span up for both these overly long books). Both featured scenes of book stealing. It sounded good, so I started shoplifting from the local Borders bookstore. The bookstore later folded and I felt like I had done my bit in their downfall. A kleptomania kick bled into some serious delusions of grandeur. Books will make you think of grand schemes like that; mania, too.

Not Well, Sure, But Just Angry

A psychiatrist I was seeing once insinuated that a famous person had secured a fairly dubious diagnosis of bipolarity – as in the fact that he was diagnosed at all – and it was one that could explain any number of felonies within a court of law, if not quite the public court of opinion. I was upset with the psychiatrist for revealing this – firstly, as a breach of doctor–patient confidentiality, and, secondly, because it revealed the fragility, and potential fictitiousness, of his own practice. It made mania co-optable to conmen, in my mind, and I wondered if I was one too – important to consider, certainly, but if I thought about it too long at this delicate stage, it would likely break me. So, I hastily put it down to famous people being megalomaniacs, not to be trusted, and walked away from sustained thought on the subject. The first psychiatrist I ever saw was a man in his late eighties – well beyond retirement age – who looked at me plainly following my short stint in his ward, and offered that I was simply 'an angry young man'. Had I invented this madness, or had I misread it, not seen the white-hot rage for what it was: legitimate and real, but not mania.

Here's Jack, the Badass

Jack Nicholson became the avatar of my manias. I would watch clips from his movies – in which he went loud and large – as a way of consolidating my own rages. There were many samples to choose from, but one, in particular, stuck. In the Hal Ashby film *The Last Detail*, Nicholson plays Signalman First Class Billy L 'Badass' Buddusky. He goes to a bar, with his colleagues, and is refused service by the barman. Things escalate from there:

SIGNALMAN FIRST CLASS BILLY L 'BADASS' BUDDUSKY: I'm going to kick your ass around the block for drill, man.

BARMAN: You try it and I'm going to call the shore patrol.

SIGNALMAN FIRST CLASS BILLY L 'BADASS' BUDDUSKY: I am the motherfucking shore patrol, motherfucker! I am the motherfucking shore patrol!

I would play the clip over and over again, going around the house repeating 'I am the motherfucking shore patrol!' During this same time, a friend mailed me a t-shirt from Bali, bought on the street, with an image of Nicholson smoking a cigar, on the front. The design was crude, but the message was received.

If You Say It, Is It So?

What evidence is there in Ben Lerner's *Leaving the Atocha Station* that the main character, in fact, does have bipolar? In the new classic, Lerner's character (and possible Lerner stand in) Adam Gordon confesses: 'I was a violent, bipolar, compulsive liar.' The novel is widely claimed to be semi-autobiographical, so what does it say about Lerner if this fact lands on one half of the fictional divide or the other? David Shields lovingly says that the book 'chronicles the endemic disease of our time: the difficulty of feeling'; is that disease bipolarity? How far can metaphor go before it loops back to reality, its starting position?

Another Theft

I walked into the university and down the hallways of the Creative Writing department, lifted the Fred Williams print straight off the wall, and promptly walked out with it. It was a reproduction, worthless really, but I wondered if anyone ever noticed it gone.

Go Fuck Yourself

One doesn't exactly wake up whistling and thinking to one-self, 'I will end this day by going to hospital' – well, not me, at least, but then the thought of a hospital stay had been loom-ing over me for weeks. I had spun out of control after an extended conflict with someone close to me and my mood was fluctuating at a rapid pace, from extremely low to a kind of excited anger. I had started smoking as a way out of the stress, and the coughs that came with the durries kept me up at night. I was popping Valium at least twice a day, proba-bly more than was recommended (it wasn't my prescription anyway). Through all of this my wife and I discussed finding a private hospital where I could get some on-hand psychiatric help. It was unaffordable and became just another mark on a long list of how mental health services in this country are hugely inaccessible.

Redacted

And I need to keep some things to myself – not just the good things. I have to withhold some of my pain too. Something happened to me during this time. It wasn't the worst thing in the world. Writing about it, however, really would be a form of petty point scoring on my part, and in the legendary words of the *Peep Show* character Mark Corrigan, 'As a petty and vindictive person I have to take extra care not to appear petty or vindictive.'

After Redacted

I texted a journo mate to see if he wanted to meet up to sink a few beers. When I walked into the pub, he was pale, and I realised quickly that he had had a worse day than mine. He had published a story detailing the suicide of a young man. As soon as the story went live, he had been on the phone to several of the parties involved, dealing with vexations of multiple verities. The emails, too, bounced up and down on his phone, and when we met, at 7.30 p.m., they showed no sign of slowing.

My mate is as good a journalist as you can get: literary, even-handed, and, above all else, a humanist seeking human truths. He had spent years writing about injustices, but was particularly well known for looking at stories of abuse, depression and inhuman government policy. He said his pallor likely came from the cumulative effect of all these stories. This latest story hit with the weight of the others behind it.

I sat and listened, did my best to counsel in my own shaky state, and drank and smoked – a whole pack in a single sitting. I called my wife to see if she could pick us up and drop us home.

The Problem with Empathy

The problem with empathy is taking on too much of the stories you hear, or letting them in too deep – namely, over-empathising, which can leave you with a hangover worse than a session of binge-drinking. In this case, I became very drunk indeed off my friend's stories and sapped up his sorrows too quickly and easily. We dropped him off out the front of his house, and he stumbled inside. When I returned home,

I slipped in my mind, and became extremely distressed – unpacking both what happened to me that day and the story of the young man's suicide. I was beyond agitated, and began to scream at my wife, 'Show them what they've done to me' over and over again, as well as beating myself on the side of the head – my preferred form of self-harm over the years. I smashed a beer bottle against our study wall, before storming into the lounge room to overturn the coffee table.

The Ride

The ambulance came soon after. My wife decided against calling the police, although hospital staff would later question that decision. I had composed myself, hiding the signs of mania that gripped me earlier, choosing to sit upright on the edge of our bed, awaiting inspection. A series of questions came from a gentle, handsome man as his colleague surveyed the scene I had left behind. I followed dutifully into the back of the ambulance, my wife sitting up the front, the warmly kind ambulance driver passing her tissues as she sobbed. As for me, I was giggling and groggily explaining what I thought had occurred, as the ambo made careful notes. An invoice for over $1000 would appear weeks later, my ambulance insurance apparently having expired.

In the Waiting Room

In the hospital waiting room, I laughed and imagined myself as some Hannibal Lecter–style creature. I had been watching clips of *The Silence of the Lambs* and the titular *Hannibal* on repeat for weeks, Anthony Hopkins' cold metallic voice calming me down, and the suggestion of there being some greater evil than myself out there easing the edges of my own perceived villainy. This is the worst kind of lived experience of pop psychology. When you're asked to explain your own inner madness, you feel the need to perform it outwardly. So, I was making crazy eyes. But I was making them as entertainment for myself and, I hoped, for my wife, to leaven the mood. We were in an emergency room after all, and were unsure of what horrors others were experiencing. There were the heavy, tired eyes of young people, surely dealing with parents' or grandparents' cancer diagnoses, or worn down from hearing the results of surgeries on the hearts and other parts of loved ones. Our experience could be a little lighter – this wasn't terminal, yet. So, I could play-act any number of lines from dark pop entertainments. Perhaps I was rehearsing for whoever would eventually come to ask me just how bad it was, and didn't want to stuff up my audition for a long stay in a psychiatric ward. My wife has often been concerned by the way I straighten up in front of health professionals – acting 'sane' in order to not cause a fuss. This would create an unnecessary barrier for receiving the treatment that I needed. I'd need to call upon fiction to show how things really were, then. Regardless, we sat for about two hours; enough time to go mad all over again.

Nurse Ratchets It Up

The nurse led me to the bed. I was surprised to get a bed. I thought I was going to get an interrogation room, like the last time I had come to a clinic due to a toxic combination of rapid thoughts and rage. The bed was comfortable enough, and it was getting late so I felt like sleeping. But there were verbal tests to do. Throughout the night I was asked to repeat the story of the preceding day four times to four different professionals – the first had been the ambulance driver, and I thought I did a very good job of it. The second was the nurse who led me to the bed, and this time it wasn't so good, as I was nodding off to sleep. The third was a stern, young, robotic doctor, with blond hair and the face of a 1980s action movie villain, of the German variety, who seemed ready to judge, not to offer any healing solutions. The hospital bed was suddenly in a court room in that telling, as he silently nodded, then asked me how many drinks I'd had. There was a sigh of relief when he left, and I wasn't sure if it was just me or the entire ward. Finally, a psychiatrist, the person we probably should have seen first, came as the hour got close to 4 a.m. and I was truly weary. Here is the thing about my mania, though – it's set off by a lack of sleep, so the fact that the people who were attempting to administer some form of care were, in fact, keeping me up until this hour, letting me have little dozes before they arrived with questions, was deeply weird. They were becoming part of the problem I was trying to get them to solve. The psychiatrist seemed kind, but she was asking incredibly blunt, almost philosophical questions, which were inappropriate for the hour. These largely had to do with whether my behaviour constituted abuse of my partner – verbal or otherwise – and while they were questions that should be asked and dealt with, looking back I don't figure them wise in the state of an acute crisis. They were reflective questions for when the storm had quietened down. It was clear that it was too early to go any deeper and I was administered a Valium and sent home. We got a cab in the early hours of the morning and collapsed in bed, bemused by the system that was supposed to be our salvage.

And Then He Hit Me, or Intended To

The young writer who, out of everyone in his generation, has played most with the idea of masculinity in Australian literature wanted to punch me in the head. His fists were curled up, and his shoulders lurched and were ready to lunge. I gave him room, told him that I loved him. I repeated, 'I love you, I love you, I love you.' I talked him down, but it took all my energy and I was anxious for days on end. I darted out of my parents' driveway in their car, and scraped the tail on a letterbox. Later, I would reflect that he too had been unstable and that I held no ill will towards him – but I would no longer talk to others who I felt had stirred him up, sent him towards me, for their own amusement. It was a dangerous game in the end.

A Final Reading

A week later I was at a reading night in Brunswick for the launch of the literary journal *The Slow Canoe*, taking the stage with five other writers who had written five short paragraphs for it. I had been asked to fill in for the poet and essayist Fiona Wright, a friend of mine, who was unable to make it down to Melbourne to read her work. I was groggy and in no good mood. People were watching out for me, but I didn't know that. I joked that I might not have been the best person to read Fiona's work – namely that I don't quite seem like a thoughtful young woman who produces some of this country's best nonfiction. But Fiona had chosen me, so I dutifully arrived

at the small warehouse space and sank a couple of beers waiting for the evening to begin. I figured I should probably read
Fiona's work at least once in my head before getting on stage
to read it aloud, so I snuck out down an alleyway and stood on
a street corner breathlessly reading the text. All seemed fine
until I hit a short piece about a friend of Fiona's who seemed
to be suffering mental ill health. I had to go over some of the
details to make sure it wasn't me (the guy in the piece had
just broken up with a girlfriend and was having breakfast
with Fiona; I hadn't broken up with anyone in five years, and
couldn't remember having breakfast with Fiona following a
break-up anyway). I realised reading something so close to
home – close to my being, as in it could be about me – might
be tough, so I recruited a friend who was also reading at the
event, to play understudy. I said I might need to call her up to
the stage if I couldn't finish reading Fiona's work:

> Daylight savings begins, its first day is glazed and
> viciously windy. I have coffee with a friend from
> my last hospitalisation, he's changing his meds this
> fortnight and not sleeping, struggling terribly as a
> result. He's dating, and that fraught combination of
> uncertainty and vulnerability that go hand-in-hand
> with going hand-in-hand with another person have
> him reeling, and I'm saddened, because the last time
> I saw him he'd been doing really well.

That was the line that broke me, 'The last time I saw him he'd
been doing really well.' I wasn't doing so well. The friend I
had asked to sub in for me if it got too much stepped forward, but through tears, I said I would finish the damn thing.

271

I ended the reading and walked out into the night air, for res-pite and a quick cigarette. I didn't want to see anyone after this, but there were friends I wanted to talk to, so I stuck it out and grinned through gritted, yellowed teeth for the rest of the night.

The Others

I meet with a friend of a friend at a local café, after she has just come out of hospital, where she had been diagnosed with bipolar for the first time. She is confused, and maybe a little scared. Afterwards, she messages me about her trials with lithium – the tremors are freaking her out. A friend of hers called me asking for advice when she was in the thick of it, and I gave what I could – care for her, tell only those you can trust, and offer her a couch and a friendly hand. Sitting over coffee, we talk and I feel like I have no more wisdom to impart – writing the book has bled me dry. I struggle with the right words. I'm not a doctor, I think. I have met a number of other writers who have also gone on to be diagnosed as manic depressive – I can relate to their experiences, just. There is, however, something so individual about the experience that it makes you shirk from any communal sharing. I feel guilty about this feeling.

Carrie Fisher at Comic-Con

At Comic-Con in San Diego, Carrie Fisher was asked by a young boy sitting in the audience to describe manic depres-sion. She replied, generously: 'It's a kind of virus of the brain. It makes you go very fast or very sad. Or both. Those are fun days. So, judgment isn't one of my big good things. But I have a good voice. I can write well. I'm not a good bicycle rider. Just like everybody else, only louder and faster and sleeps more.'

I Can Write Well

I can say that I have a good voice and I can write. I genuinely think I can, and it may, indeed, spring from some inner well of mania within me, but at least I have tried to put it to good use, to say to you, reading this, that this was my life, or at least part of it. From here I can hope to act a little better – to be a little more humane when I'm less than human. I can hope to slow down when I am going so fast, when I am not such a good rider of these rapids.

This Book

And you see this book here? I'm going to teach you to speak my language with this book.

AUTHOR'S NOTE

The opening line of 'Rapid thought generator' is directly lifted from the first line of Jonathan Lethem's *The Disappointment Artist*. Lethem, no stranger to quotation and appropriation (see *The Ecstasy of Influence*), would not mind, I am certain. The quote is repeated in the chapter on Carrie Fisher for good measure.

The quote from Kanye West on *The Ellen DeGeneres Show* came from an episode dated 19 May 2016 and was widely shared on YouTube. I subjected myself willingly to transcribing it in full.

Parts of this book have previously been published in different forms, and under different titles, in *Meanjin*, *The Rumpus*, the *Sydney Morning Herald*, *Seizure* magazine, and *Writers Victoria*. My sincere thanks go to the editors of those publications.

WORKS CONSULTED

Books

Adler, Renata, *Speedboat*, Random House, New York, 1976

American Psychiatric Association, *The Diagnostic and Statistic Manual of Mental Disorders, Fifth Edition (DSM-5)*, American Psychiatric Association, Washington, 2013

Atlas, James, *Delmore Schwartz: The Life of an American Poet*, Farrar, Straus and Giroux, New York, 1977

Bailey, Blake, *A Tragic Honesty: The Life and Work of Richard Yates*, Picador, New York, 2003

Bellow, Saul, *The Adventures of Augie March*, The Viking Press, New York, 1953

_____ *Seize the Day*, Weidenfeld and Nicolson, London, 1957

_____ *Herzog*, The Viking Press, New York, 1964

_____ *Humboldt's Gift*, The Viking Press, New York, 1975

Berger, John, *Ways of Seeing*, British Broadcasting Corporation and Penguin Books, London, 1972

Berryman, John, *Recovery*, University of Minnesota Press edition, Minneapolis, 2016

Broyard, Anatole, *Intoxicated by My Illness: and Other Writings on Life and Death*, Fawcett Columbine, New York, 1993

Caramagno, Thomas C, *The Flight of the Mind*, University of California Press, Berkeley, 1992

Casey, Nell (editor), *The Journals of Spalding Gray*, Knopf, New York, 2011

Custance, John, *Wisdom, Madness and Folly: The Philosophy of a Lunatic*, Victor Gollancz, London, 1951

Demastes, William W, *Spalding Gray's America*, Limelight Editions, New York, 2008

Didion, Joan, *The White Album*, Farrar, Straus and Giroux, New York, 1979

Duke, Patty and Hochman, Gloria, *A Brilliant Madness: Living with Manic-Depressive Illness*, Bantam Books, New York, 1992

Dyer, Geoff, *Out of Sheer Rage*, Picador, London, 1997

Exley, Frederick, *A Fan's Notes*, Vintage Contemporaries Edition, NewYork, 1988

Fisher, Carrie, *Postcards from the Edge*, Simon & Schuster, New York, 1987
_____ *The Best Awful*, Simon & Schuster, New York, 2003
_____ *Wishful Drinking*, Simon & Schuster, New York, 2008
_____ *Shockaholic*, Simon & Schuster, New York, 2011
_____ *The Princess Diarist*, Blue Rider Press, New York, 2016
Fitzgerald, F Scott, *The Crack-Up*, New Directions, New York, 1945
Flaherty, Alice W, *The Midnight Disease: The Drive to Write, Writer's Block, and the Creative Brain*, Mariner Books, New York, 2005
Gray, Spalding, *Swimming to Cambodia: The Collected Works of Spalding Gray*, Picador, London, 1987
_____ *Monster in a Box*, Pan Books, London, 1991
_____ *Impossible Vacation*, Picador, London, 1993
Greenberg, Michael, *Hurry Down Sunshine*, Bloomsbury Publishing, London, 2009
Griffiths, Jay, *Tristimania: A Diary of Manic Depression*, Hamish Hamilton, London, 2016
Hamilton, Craig, with Jameson, Neil, *Broken Open*, Bantam Books, Sydney, 2005
Hardwick, Elizabeth, *Sleepless Nights*, Random House, New York, 1979
Healy, David, *Mania: A Short History of Bipolar Disorder*, John Hopkins University Press, Baltimore, 2008
Hinshaw, Stephen, *Another Kind of Madness: A Journey Through the Stigma and Hope of Mental Illness*, St. Martins Press, New York, 2017
Hornbacher, Marya, *Madness: A Bipolar Life*, Fourth Estate, London, 2008
Jefferson, Margo, *On Michael Jackson*, Vintage Books, New York, 2007
Johns, Andrew, with Cadigan, Neil, *The Two of Me*, HarperCollins, Sydney, 2007
Koestenbaum, Wayne, *Humiliation*, Picador, New York, 2011
Kraepelin, Emil, *Manic-depressive Insanity and Paranoia*, ES Livingstone, Edinburgh, 1921
Leader, Darian, *Strictly Bipolar*, Penguin Books, London, 2013
Leader, Zachary, *The Life of Saul Bellow: To Fame and Fortune 1915–1964*, Knopf, New York, 2015
Lerner, Ben, *Leaving the Atocha Station*, Coffee House Press, Minneapolis, 2011
Lethem, Jonathan, *The Disappointment Artist*, Vintage Contemporaries Edition, New York, 2005
Malcolm, Janet, *The Silent Woman: Sylvia Plath & Ted Hughes*, Knopf, New York, 1993
Martin, Emily, *Bipolar Expeditions: Mania and Depression in American Culture*, Princeton University Press, Princeton, 2007
Max, DT, *Every Love Story Is a Ghost Story: A Life of David Foster Wallace*, Penguin, New York, 2012
Meyers, Jeffrey, *Manic Power: Robert Lowell and his Circle*, Arbor House, New York, 1987

Works consulted

Michaels, Leonard, *Sylvia*, Farrar, Straus and Giroux, New York, 1990
Mikics, David, *Bellow's People: How Saul Bellow Made Life into Art*, WW Norton & Company, New York, 2016
Prichard, James Cowles, *A Treatise on Insanity and Other Disorders Affecting the Mind*, Sherwood, Gilbert and Piper, London, 1835
Redfield Jamison, Kay, *Touched with Fire: Manic-Depressive Illness and the Artistic Temperament*, Free Press Paperback Edition, New York, 1994
_____ *An Unquiet Mind*, Picador, London, 1996
_____ *Exuberance: The Passion for Life*, Vintage Books, New York, 2005
_____ *Robert Lowell: Setting the River on Fire*, Knopf, New York, 2017
Richards, Kate, *Madness: A Memoir*, Penguin Books Australia, Melbourne, 2013
Schwartz, Delmore, *In Dreams Begin Responsibilities*, New Directions, New York, 1978 (first published 1938)
Shields, David, *How Literature Saved My Life*, Knopf, New York, 2013
Simpson, Eileen, *Poets in Their Youth*, Farrar, Straus and Giroux, New York, 1990
Sontag, Susan, *Illness as Metaphor*, Farrar, Straus and Giroux, New York, 1978
Styron, William, *Darkness Visible*, Random House, New York, 1990
Whybrow, Peter C, *A Mood Apart: Depression, Mania, and Other Afflictions of the Self*, Basic Books, New York, 2015

Films

The Last Detail, dir. Hal Ashby (1973)
A Woman Under the Influence, dir. John Cassavetes (1974)
Star Wars, dir. George Lucas (1977)
Swimming to Cambodia, dir. Jonathan Demme (1987)
Terrors of Pleasure, dir. Thomas Schlamme (1988)
Mr Jones, dir. Mike Figgis (1993)
Crumb, dir. Terry Zwigoff (1994)
Magnolia, dir. Paul Thomas Anderson (1999)
Punch-Drunk Love, dir. Paul Thomas Anderson (2002)
I Heart Huckabees, dir. David O Russell (2004)
The Assassination of Jesse James by the Coward Robert Ford, dir. Andrew Dominik (2007)
Michael Clayton, dir. Tony Gilroy (2007)
There Will Be Blood, dir. Paul Thomas Anderson (2007)
The Informant!, dir. Steven Soderbergh (2009)
The Master, dir. Paul Thomas Anderson (2012)
Inherent Vice, dir. Paul Thomas Anderson (2014)
Infinitely Polar Bear, dir. Maya Forbes (2014)
Love & Mercy, dir. Bill Pohlad (2014)
Touched with Fire, dir. Paul Dalio (2015)
A Bigger Splash, dir. Luca Guadagnino (2015)

A Quiet Dream, dir. Zhang Lu (2016)
Lion, dir. Garth Davis (2016)
Bright Lights: Starring Carrie Fisher and Debbie Reynolds, dir. Alex Bloom and
    Fisher Stevens (2017)

Articles

Beck, Taylor, 'Kin By Mania: The Bond I Feel With Other Bipolar People Is
    Inexplicable', *Huffington Post*, 21 May 2017
Cadwalladr, Carole, 'Jason Russell: Kony2012 and the search for truth',
    Guardian, 3 March 2013
Cole, Teju, 'The White-Savior Industrial Complex', *Atlantic*, 21 March 2012
Diski, Jenny, 'Having Half the Fun', *London Review of Books*, May 1996
Du Bois, William, 'Books of the Times', *New York Post*, 23 July 1945
Dyer, Geoff, 'Reader's Block', *LA Weekly*, 1 March 2000
Invisible Children, 'Recap: Jason Russell on *Oprah*', 8 October 2012
Lehmann, John, 'Time for Troubled Andrew Johns to "Man Up"', *Daily
    Telegraph*, 12 May 2013
Leitan, Nuwan D, 'The Self in Bipolar Disorder', *The Self in Understanding
    and Treating Psychological Disorders*, Cambridge University Press,
    Cambridge, 2016
Lowe, Jaime, 'I Don't Believe in God but I Do Believe in Lithium', *New York
    Times*, 25 June 2015
McClean, Krit, 'A Manic Episode Led Me to Strip Naked in Times Square',
    New York Post, 6 August 2016
Milsom, Rosemarie, 'Matthew Newton's Struggle with Bipolar Disorder',
    Newcastle Herald, 13 April 2012
Muscat, Kat, 'Triangles: The Holey Trinity of Possible BPD', *Stilts*, August
    2014
Nededog, Jethro, 'Kony 2012 Filmmaker Jason Russell's Wife Addresses His
    Flip Out', *Hollywood Reporter*, 21 March 2012
Newman, Judith, '"Spalding Gray" the Color? It's a Long Story', *New York
    Times*, 28 December 2017
Ohlson, Kristin, 'Unravelling Man', *Aeon Magazine*, April 2014
Phillips, Carl, 'On Restlessness', *New England Review*, vol. 30, no. 1, 2009
Sacks, Oliver, 'The Catastrophe: Spalding Gray's Brain Injury', *New Yorker*,
    27 April 2015
Wickman, Forrest, 'Naked Lunch', *Slate*, 29 May 2012
Williams, Alex, 'Vanishing Act', *New York Magazine*, 2 February 2004
Wright, Fiona, 'Spring Diary', *Five by Five* published by *Slow Canoe*, 2017
Wright, Tom, 'Artists Behind Splendour's Controversial "Sad Kanye"
    Artwork Respond To Criticism', *Music Feeds*, 2 June 2017

ACKNOWLEDGMENTS

What are acknowledgments for exactly? Someone remind me, because this whole book would, hopefully, stand as the sincerest form of acknowledgment possible – a testament to those who have supported me, and, frankly, on so many levels, kept me alive. This includes a core group of family, friends and colleagues. To my immediate family, particularly my parents, Kim and Steve B Cool, you lived through more of this than you should have, but did so with much grace, dignity and integrity.

I dedicate this book to the loving memories of both Kat Muscat and Miss Helen, dear friends both of whom provided much kinship in discussing issues relating to mental health during the time I knew them, and who both departed this timeline far too soon.

I also wish to extend a particular thanks to Rebecca Giggs for introducing me to Carl Phillips' wonderful essay 'On Restlessness', which gave me the epigraph of this book and guided much of its thinking and, also, for posting me a copy of Alice W Flaherty's excellent *The Midnight Disease* after collegial conversations about where my writing was heading, knowing very well that this book might result. May every writer have friends and colleagues as engaged in your work as I have been lucky enough to acquire over the years. Thank you to Martin McKenzie-Murray, Nick Tapper, Fiona Wright and Khalid

Warsame for generous conversations around this book. And thank you to Alan 'Weeds' Weedon for riding in the passenger seat next to me during my most eccentric of travels. I don't wish to thank anyone else by name here – in the real fear of being caught out forgetting others – but you all know who you are, and you know how much your help meant to me along the way.

This book simply would not exist without the foresight and guidance of its publisher, Phillipa McGuinness, who saw promise in the tiniest of fragments supplied and convinced me that it was a worthwhile endeavour. This book owes much to the seminal editing skills of Jocelyn Hungerford (to whom I promise to never use the word seminal again). The editing and publishing process not only made the book better, both brought out the best in me, within a work that required so much to be put on the line.

Writing in the era of late capitalism is often a filthy, degrading act. In all truth, it is financially unviable. The largest thanks, then – for supporting the writing and research time necessary to bring this work to completion – must go to my wife-in-crime, Brigid 'Bridie' Mullane. This book simply could not be in your hands without her economic support and daily dedication to my wellbeing. I hope I can pay you back some day soon, Bridie. Yet as we well know, your love is a quantity that exists free of market values, as it goes to the heart of what it means to be human. And if this book has any life to it at all – indeed, if I have any life at all – it is because of you.

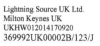